I0505749

Erasing Autism:

The Spectrum Balance® Protocol

By: Dr. Shauna K. Young, PhD, CTN

Sky UnLimited, LLC

Prímum non nocere

Copyright © 2015 by Dr Shauna K. Young, Phd, CTN

All rights reserved. No part of this publication may be reproduced, distributed, or transmitted in any form or by any means, including photocopying, recording, or other electronic or mechanical methods, without the prior written permission of the publisher, except in the case of brief quotations embodied in critical reviews and certain other noncommercial uses permitted by copyright law.

Although the stories contained herein are real, specific names and identifying details have been changed to protect the privacy of individuals. The information provided herein is only intended as anecdotal rather than advisory, and cannot substitute for the advice of a professional. Nothing herein is to be construed as an attempt to offer or render a professional medical or nutritional opinion, which cannot be done effectively without individualized consultation. Please consult with a physician before beginning any dietary or exercise regimen. Reliance on any information provided is solely at your own risk.

This book is offered for informational, educational and entertainment purposes only. As Dr. Shauna Young is not a medical doctor (M.D.), she does not give out what is legally referred to as "medical advice". If you have any known medical conditions, please consult with your doctor before making any significant changes in your diet, supplementation, medications, exercise or other lifestyle aspects.

ISBN-13: 978-1507535097
ISBN-10: 1507535090

Library of Congress Control Number:
CreateSpace, North Charleston, SC

This book is dedicated:

To all the amazing families who have traveled from across the country and across the world to my office, bringing their children with trust and hope in their hearts and willing to try one more thing…

To all those who could not make it in to my office, but had the wherewithal to take on the Spectrum Balance Protocol themselves at home in the hope of benefiting their children…

To the wonderful group of neurodevelopmentalists who recommend this Protocol to the kids they work with in the hopes that it will cement their work with them…

To the kind and generous people who have donated their hard earned funds to The NoHarm Foundation in the hopes that it will benefit even more children…

Hope. It was in their hearts…

Now, hope is on your plate…

About the Author

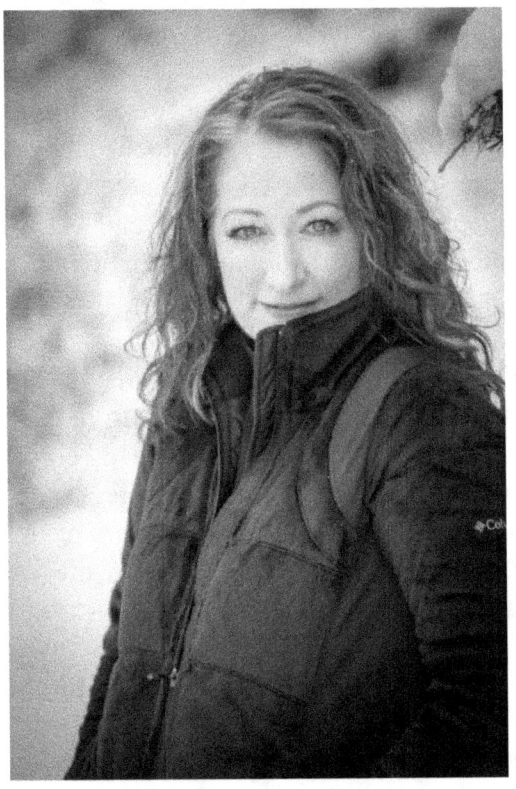

Shauna K. Young
Ph.D., CTN, CBS, OSJ

    Dr. Shauna Young, is the owner and Medical Director of the Assertive Wellness Research Center of Durango, CO, which first opened its doors in 2001. To date, her center has had seen thousands of clients who have had the confidence to travel from every U.S. State and even several foreign countries based almost exclusively on referrals from other practitioners and satisfied clients.

In 2005, after four years of clinical observations and experience, Shauna began specific research regarding her theorized negative effects of excess and stored manganese on the human neurological and sensory input systems and its possible symptomatic connections to Autism and other neurological, learning and behavioral disorders in both children and adults. The unique success of this clinical research, originally referred to as "The Popeye Protocol" and currently as the "Spectrum Balance® Protocol", led to her receiving Distinguished Awards of Excellence in both May of 2006 and May of 2007 from the internationally-recognized Global Foundation for Integrative Medicine.

Shauna holds a Bachelor of Science Degree in Natural Sciences and was awarded a PhD in Natural Sciences from the University of Natural Medicine in Santa Fe, New Mexico. In February of 2008 she was also knighted into the international Sovereign Medical Order of the Knights Hospitaller in recognition of the unique impact of her work with Autism and for positively advancing the field of natural medicine in general.

Shauna serves as the Chief Medical Advisor for the NoHarm Foundation (www.noharmfoundation.org), a Colorado not-for-profit organization formed with the primary goal of releasing this vastly important information with the intent of ushering in a new paradigm in research and providing real help for countless suffering children and adults. This information to date has been downloaded and utilized at no cost to families living in more than 67 countries.

Her very well reviewed first book "If Naturopaths are Quacks, Then I Guess I'm a Duck" was published in April of 2012. She is currently an internationally recognized speaker and educator, and is working on her third book.

Disclosure and Disclaimer

Although the stories contained herein are real, specific names and identifying details have been changed to protect the privacy of individuals. The information provided herein is only intended as anecdotal rather than advisory, and cannot substitute for the advice of a professional. Nothing herein is to be construed as an attempt to offer or render a professional medical or nutritional opinion, which cannot be done effectively without individualized consultation. Please consult with a physician before beginning any dietary or exercise regimen. Reliance on any information provided is solely at your own risk.

This book is offered for informational, educational and entertainment purposes only. As Dr. Shauna Young is not a medical doctor (M.D.), she does not give out what is legally referred to as "medical advice". If you have any known medical conditions, please consult with your doctor before making any significant changes in your diet, supplementation, medications, exercise or other lifestyle aspects.

So much for the legal part. On to the book...

The Basics of the "Paleo Diet":

The diet featured in this book, The Spectrum Balance® Protocol, is NOT the standard Paleo diet. It is a targeted Protocol meant to correct a mineral imbalance in the brain that will be explained. It is however, by all definition, a Paleo diet.

"Paleo" is short for "Paleolithic" and represents the blossoming and derivative dietary philosophies that have primarily resulted from the initial theories and work of Loren Cordain, PhD. There is excellent and building evidence that mankind's transitions away from Paleo "Caveman-type" diets, initially beginning with the current Neolithic period considered to by around 10,000 years ago, have not only led to largely different food mix and sources of "modern" nutrition, but have greatly contributed to much of the malnutrition and disease that we see today. It seems that our human bodies just may neither have been designed nor have even yet adequately adapted to eat diets that more modern cultures have found through agriculture to be most manageable, economical and convenient.

Following Paleo practices, you eat meats of all types, vegetables, fruit, good fats and a few nuts. No grains, no legumes, no overly pro-cessed foods (like soda, breads, etc.) and limited or no dairy (based on sensitivity). Portion size and even calorie counting is far less im-portant than the simple exclusion of the problematic foods. I like the fact that even though you'll find many references to Paleo "diet(s)", this truly represents a lifestyle eating philosophy that is in no way suggested as some short-term fix for weight loss alone that you'll soon discard and want to return to your old eating habits. Once you go Paleo, you'll want to stay with it for life.

In 2012, "Paleo Diet" did not even hit the top ten of dietary terms used in a Google search. By 2013, "Paleo Diet" was the number one dietary term used in Google searches.

Would you like to guess where it was for 2014? Still number one. If it ain't broke, don't fix it…

Contents

Contents

CHAPTER ONE

Ground Zero: Jay's Story

June 15, 2005 was a Wednesday much like any other, or so I thought. That afternoon, a harassed mom brought in her three-year-old son with the ill-defined hope that I could do "something" to help him. Eight months earlier, he had received the diagnosis, or *sentence* as it felt to her, of "autism" and in keeping with the current paradigm of "no known cause, no known treatment, no known cure" had been given no hope of making any significant changes for him. The young family did not have a large income at its disposal and was feeling very adrift and without options. Since I had worked successfully with some odd health issues recently with one of Jay's cousins, his mom had brought him in more on a basis of hope than of expectation.

Although I wasn't sure what the "something" I might be able to do would look like, I was willing to try. This was the first autistic child I had ever worked with and was eager to see what I could discern. Testing him with my bio-feedback system was certainly an experience I will never forget. Even with his mother constantly chasing after him saying "Jay, no!" "Jay, come here!" "Jay, stop touching that!" he was still making a wreck of my office, charging around, touching and smelling everything like a little wild animal, making odd screeching sounds, and even taking a bite out of one of my plants! Not more than a few minutes into the process my head was ringing not only from his yelps, screaming and crying, but from the pleading of his besieged mother. To make matters even worse, the poor kid was also terrified of me, which seemed strange because kids usually like me. His mother, in his defense, explained that he was terrified of all female doctors because of multiple incidents with a woman doctor who was very rough with him and had even performed a minor surgical procedure (snipping off a piece of fore-skin) on him without the benefit of anesthesia. The doctor told the horrified mom when this happened that "Autistic kids don't feel very much." Do you think she wondered why the boy was screaming his brains out if it didn't hurt? It was no wonder the kid was scared of me or any doctor for that matter!

One of the many reasons that the diagnosis of autism is so dif-ficult to deal with is because it is a permanent brand not only on a child but on the whole family. This little guy had started out life well, and at the age of one he seemed more advanced than slow. He walked at an early age, and had been adding words to his vocabu-lary on a nearly daily basis. This all halted abruptly from one day to the next after he went in for some routine childhood vaccinations. The day after he had his DPT, MMR and HIB vaccines, he spiked a fever and was exhibiting flu-like symptoms. The doctors assured his mother that this was a "normal" reaction to the vaccines, but things with him were anything but normal afterwards. From that point on he never spoke another word, and a few months later the diagnosis was in. Autism. The relation to the vaccines was determined to be "coincidental."

The story about the doctor, however, is what first struck me about his "autism." Autistic children in general are nearly completely indifferent to their surroundings, including a marked indifference to other people. Why then would he only react with fear to *female* doc-tors, and not to males? How would he even recognize that a person was a doctor in the first place? I don't wear a white coat or any other identifying "doctor" paraphernalia, and my office looks pretty much like any other office. It even lacks that distinctive "doctor's office smell" that so intimidates many of us. So, if he had been exhibiting the usual detachment from others that most autistic children do, why would he even make the distinction? This made me look for more examples in the same vein.

His behavior did exhibit plenty of consistencies with autism. The frequent outbursts and tantrums, the complete lack of intelligible (or even unintelligible) speech, and most noticeably, his incredibly over-reactive senses. However, his unusual male/female/doctor distinction was enough to pique my interest and encourage me to seek more inconsistencies.

As the appointment went on there were plenty to choose from. Typical autistic children are usually quite indifferent to their surroundings; the very basis of autism is that they "live in their own world." Jay, on the other hand, was assiduously investigating everything he could get his hands on: smelling, feeling, and even tasting, once taking a bite out of a large plant in my office! He played effectively and for a long period of time with a toy that often confuses adults. His motor skills were excellent. Most unusually he watched me like a cat, often making long-term eye contact with me. He showed plenty of diverse emotions by both cuddling with his mother and then showing clearly that he was terrified of me. Despite his erratic behavior, *none of rest of this fit with the accepted pattern of autism.* Though extremely heightened sensitivity to touch, light, smell and noise is consistent with autism, it struck me that even though the physical touch from his mother seemed to hurt him, *he kept returning to her when feeling the most frightened.* It was as if even though it hurt him the comfort was worth the pain. Again, not the uncaring and "in-their-own-world" behavior of autism. I could see I needed to be on my toes with this one.

In the course of the assessment process, in which I used a non-invasive type of bio-resonant/ bio-feedback computer interfaced equipment, one word kept popping up repeatedly -- manganese. I didn't give it much thought the first few times it showed up, since mineral,

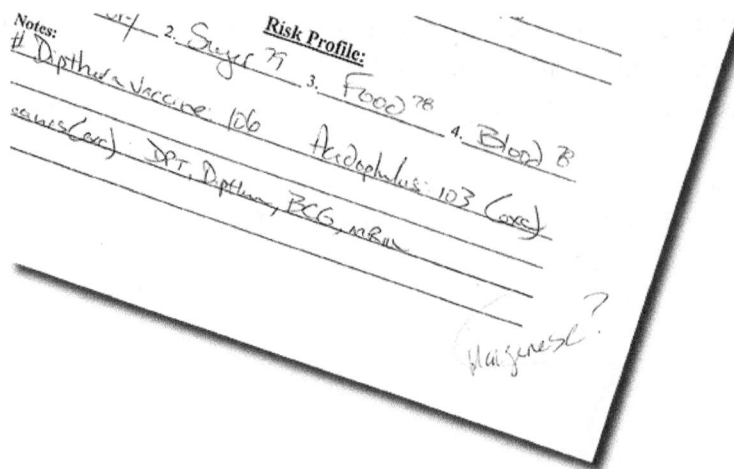

enzyme and other nutrient names often cross the screen. After re-peating itself several times however, I wrote it down with a question mark as a note on Jay's test sheet.

Normally, manganese is one of those nutrients you don't have to give a lot of thought to, as the body usually maintains it on its own. Generally, there will only be a mere 12-20 mg stored in the body at any given time. Manganese is a type of naturally occurring metal that is found in several different kinds of rocks. Referred to as the "brain mineral," it is important to the utilization of all the mental capacities and functions, as well as in the formation of tendons and ligaments, and in maintaining the structural integrity of the lining of various organs. Obviously, the "brain mineral" idea caught my atten-tion, but strangely, the signs of manganese deficiency, such as, carpal tunnel, deafness, tendon weakness and retarded growth rate did not seem to apply. Huh.

After the family left my office, the word "manganese" continued to distract me. Enough so that after office hours I pulled out Jay's chart and went over it again and again. Something was bothering me; I just couldn't put my finger on what it was. I looked for the small things in his chart that sometimes get overlooked in the hectic confines of a first appointment, especially with a kid charging around eating my plants.

When I asked if he had any allergies, his mother said that he did not, but noted that, "He throws up soy and blueberries." Looking up soy and blueberries in a nutritional handbook, I found they are both excellent sources...of manganese. Further investigation revealed that manganese excess is known to inhibit iron absorption, and Jay had exhibited many low-iron symptoms. It was all starting to make sense. This wasn't a manganese *deficiency*. This was a manganese surplus!

Armed with standard nutritional handbooks, I began searching for any problems associated with manganese excess, but I found very little information. So I turned next to the internet and after a few preliminary searches found something very interesting. After getting the wording just right on a search engine I managed to find several articles that addressed a condition called "Manganese Madness." According to numerous studies I located, the primary site of collection for manganese toxicity, *regardless of the source of exposure*, is the basal ganglia; a mass of nervous tissue that is nestled within the cerebral hemispheres. This cause-and-effect of excess manganese was first revealed by an English physician who noted all the way back in 1837 that some workers in a local manganese mine appeared "lethargic and their faces unexpressive." Since neurological textbooks identify manganese as a neurotoxic metal, and as a result of his research, the disease of "Manganism" was coined by the turn of the 20th century.

There wasn't much information to be found, but according to what I could find on "Manganism," this disease that struck manganese miners exposed to toxic dust appeared to cause symptoms of "emotional liability, irrationality, hallucinations and impulsivity." Chronic exposure led to "muscular weakness, ataxia, tremor, immobile facial expressions, and extreme speech disturbances." These symptoms, which sounded a lot like Parkinson's in adults, sounded suspiciously like autism in a child to me. More digging revealed that other very common symptoms of manganese excess can be speech difficulties and extreme reactions to sensory input: light, touch, smell and sound. *Aha!* Now I was getting somewhere.

The more research I dug up, the more fascinating and clear it became to me: *This was a manganese excess, not a lack, that might be behind Jay's symptoms.* Every report I could find described it perfectly! Something that might be encountered as "problems in speech" to an adult could well be perceived as an insurmountable obstacle to a child barely more than a year old. And his most important symptom, the overwhelming nature of his sensory input, was described in detail in each and every report. Limiting and annoying to an adult, I could completely see how terrifying it would be to such a little child.

The one thing my research did not reveal anything about was how to correct this excess. Could there be a way to somehow counter the manganese imbalance and thereby halt these disastrous effects? Was this the "something" his mother had hoped for? My hunting through medical research papers revealed no information on the topic. Given the complete lack of guidance or suggestions, I fell back on the number one tool available to a naturopath -- my common sense. If excess manganese can inhibit iron absorption, it made perfect sense to me that additional iron could possibly defeat and balance the excess manganese. It was worth a shot!

After running a quick check of the readily available foods that are highest in iron, I made the rash decision to call his mother. I was incredibly psyched about this idea and wanted to fill her in as soon as possible. She was rather surprised to hear from me, especially since it was around 9:00 pm, and I desperately hoped she wasn't going to think I was completely crazy for suggesting what I was about to tell her. I described the course I'd followed on this, and the results of the research I'd done. Then I told her my wild idea: Maybe if we loaded Jay up with dietary iron it could possibly work to overload the manganese and possibly restore the balance, which hopefully could reduce some of the sensory overload symptoms. Things got pretty quiet for a moment while she considered what I was saying, and I held my breath hoping she'd agree to try it.

Her first question concerned how to get all the iron into him. Exhaling, I suggested a list of foods that highlighted meats, spinach, dried apricots, black cherries, and a few other high-iron foods, stressing the fact that raw was the best way for him to eat the fruits and vegetables. I also reminded her to load his diet as much as she could with good fats; especially olive oil and butter. Her worry, which I would begin hearing constantly from this point on, was whether he would willingly eat these foods I suggested. "Don't all kids hate spinach?" We discussed a few food ideas and she assured me that she'd do her best, as by now she was growing a little excited by this crazy idea herself. I further suggested that she let him play with his food, eat with his hands, whatever it took. I concluded the call by asking that she keep me in the loop about his progress.

When I hung up the phone, I looked once more at what I had written in Jay's chart. One little notation, "manganese," followed by a question mark. I had no idea at the time that one little word notation would change so many lives, including mine.

Ten days after his original appointment, nine days on the high-iron protocol, Jay's mom called me to give me a progress report. First of all, to her surprise, he was absolutely loving the diet. She described him as "eating like a horse" and happily scarfing down all the veggies and iron-rich foods I had recommended. Once a picky eater, he was now looking forward to mealtimes. As I had suggested, she was letting him play with his food, eat with his hands, whatever, as long as he ate it. In something that seemed strange at that moment, that would actually come to be a norm in time, he was consuming raw spinach with gusto, even carrying the bag around and eating it with both hands "like potato chips." I asked if anything in his behavior had changed, and she gave her report. Already, in only nine days, he was slightly less sensitive to light and touch, and had stopped smelling everything "like a puppy dog."

Throughout our entire conversation, there was an undertone of ... something. She sounded excited, which I could understand, but there was something else. Finally I asked, "Is there something else? Any other changes?"

This was the question she was waiting for and sprung her news on me. "Just one -- he started to talk!"

CHAPTER TWO

The Perfect Storm

Two months after his original appointment, Jay and his mother came in with some truly wonderful news. After some new testing, Jay had been "reclassified" by his doctor as "not autistic" and he was starting pre-school in the coming semester. They had found him a therapist to help him catch up on his speech and he was progressing very quickly. Less than three months into my work with him, I discharged him from having to see me regularly; with my only dietary recommendations being that he stay off breads and cereals, and to be mindful of how much of the most manganese-rich foods he had in his diet.

The fact that Jay actually liked the diet is a point that has come up over and over again. In my many years of experience with this I have found that what people think children like, and what they actually do like, are two different things. Most people seem to think that kids "need" things like cookies, sugary cereals, toaster waffles and macaroni and cheese. Things that are referred to -- even on restaurant menus -- as "kid's foods." What I've found to be true is that kids like the same thing their parents do and if that's what winds up on the dining room table, that's what they'll eat. I once had a six-year-old who, when I told his mom they no longer needed to strictly be on the Protocol, leapt out of his chair and said, "I can still have salmon and mango's, right?"

As you can imagine after the spectacular results with my first autistic child, I dug into this idea with a vengeance. What had started more as hopeful interest was now becoming obsessive. What if it would work on others? What if I could effect this kind of change in even five percent of autism cases? With the ever-escalating number of autism cases and other ASDs even that small percentage would amount to a lot of kids!

My next major area of exploration was -- where did such a little kid obtain so much manganese? Most of the research I'd been able to find was on people with obvious explanations of where the manganese had come from, such as manganese miners.

Further research turned up some likely suspects. Since Jay had been fed a soy-based baby formula, I started there. As it turns out, soy-based baby formulas can contain 200 times the amount of manganese that is naturally contained in human breast milk. That kind of overwhelming overdose could wreak havoc on a developing brain! A paper I'd found from a London hospital had discovered that even manganese concentrations that were considered "safe" by government standards could be attributed to causing brain damage after feeding periods of only a few months.

People seem to like to think that there is some "one cause" of any disease or disorder and want to point the finger of blame at that one source, but in the course of my over a decade of practice I have rarely found that to be true. Whether someone is suffering from autism or fibromyalgia it usually involves some sort of "perfect storm" of circumstances instead of any one factor that creates the problem. The same thing holds true here, and as I did more and more research, the sources of manganese began to get overwhelming. It wasn't just the soy formula at all. There are environmental causes, water contamination, IV nutrition being fed to premature babies, pineapple, blueberries and other common foods are loaded with it; baby foods, teething biscuits, and one of the biggest culprits: vitamins. If you or anyone in your family is taking multivitamins, you may want to check the bottles for manganese. You might be surprised by what you find! With all these sources of manganese, you wouldn't think it would come as such a shock to me that I started seeing adults with high manganese as well.

What was surprising was to see how differently the same problem source was manifesting in different people. In addition to children who were on the autism spectrum, I was now seeing adults who had received diagnoses of schizophrenia, bipolar disorder, Parkinson's and Alzheimer's as well as the more nebulous, but common, lack of focus or "I think I'm losing my mind" complaint. Further, uncannily, I was observing the almost identical nature of what I had come to think of as my "markers" in every affected person regardless of his or her age. And although the results are slower in a larger person, and one more likely to cheat on the diet, we were still seeing the same positive results from the diet in adults as we were in children.

Because of it's early use of olive oil and raw spinach, our little joke in the office was calling this ever-evolving dietary change "The Popeye Protocol." So you can imagine our surprise when we turned up a strange and very jarring little fact: Spinach, one of our "hero foods" thus far, is just as good a source of manganese as it is of iron! Talk about an "oh crap" moment! This little fact became known in my office as "The Spinach Paradox" and both I and my staff began tearing into this one like crazy. Since both iron and manganese are present in spinach and yet the undeniable fact is that it had already worked, that meant that it wasn't just they were getting excess manganese. There had to be something inhibiting the bio-availability of the iron.

Enter the missing link. Paleo!

"Paleo" at the time was either an emerging science or the latest fad diet, depending on who you spoke to. It was far from the massive, nearly mainstream movement that it is today, but at least there was some research that I could get my hands on. And what I found spoke volumes to me. Because of the vast amount of sources of manganese overload, we originally felt it was simply that: Too much manganese. It would not be for a few years later when we realized what I now consider to be the primary and underestimated culprit in the formation of this imbalance of iron and manganese. It is the dietary consumption of phytic acid salts known as phytates. Phytates were unmasked to be the anti-nutrients that were robbing these peoples diets of their iron, and the "Paleo people" were all over it.

Because phytates are found in grains, legumes, seeds, and pretty much everything people usually eat for breakfast, it now made sense. This went a long way towards explaining to me why autism seemed to be striking across the board; whether they were eating the typical SAD breakfast of sugary cereal or toast, or eating what was considered a "healthy" diet with organic food and lots of "healthy whole grains." I have seen children who manifested symptoms after a vaccine, or after being fed formulas, but I've also seen it in kids who were breast-fed exclusively and had no vaccines.

For the record I should state here that although I am not a fan of vaccines, I don't think that they are the "one cause" of this massive rise in children being affected with ASDs. No, there had to be a bigger reason.

As it turns out, the phytates contained in these foods were tightly binding to calcium, magnesium, zinc, and for my purposes - iron. So nearly everything that most people are used to eating for breakfast is causing their iron and many other necessary minerals to simply flush out without being utilized. While this causes a wide variety of problems, it also leaves receptor sites in the brain wide open for business for available manganese, since there is insufficient iron to compete for the same site. **There is well documented research and evidence**

that in the case of insufficient iron and surplus manganese, brain transport mechanisms will resort to substituting manganese in brain receptor sites that are intended to function with iron.

Although the Spectrum Balance® Protocol would be considered to be a "Paleo" diet (since it eliminates phytates) it is still very important to understand that it is not the classic Paleo diet that has now been adopted by millions. Those diets still allow foods that even though they are healthy, they are too high in manganese to be usable in the Spectrum Balance® Protocol. It is vital to understand that this diet specifically addresses the iron/manganese imbalance that is causing the high sensory input that is at the basis of the autism and autism spectrum disorder symptoms.

My original hope that this Protocol could possibly help in even five percent of autism cases, was now looking like much, much more. And more than just autism.

CHAPTER THREE

An Introduction to the Case Studies

Believe it or not, the hardest part of writing this book was selecting the case studies. After many editorial cuts our "short list" was still over 70 cases! With so many to choose from it turned into a matter of "which of the miracles do we leave out!" But in order for you to be able to actually lift this book, we had to leave the vast majority of them out.

Here, we ended up presenting case studies that cover a wide base of diagnoses, symptoms, ages, family dynamics and outcomes. And while I have worked with many adults with this Protocol, we focused this time exclusively on the kids. I will ask that you please resist the temptation to scan through and just look for the one condition you are interested in. And through reading all case studies here, you will begin to see a clear pattern; you may recognize one element your case has with one child and family, and another in another situation, and so on. You will see how disparate situations all have the same positive outcome: A happier, healthier, and responsive child.

Remember that the doctors and therapists your kids are being diagnosed by are all *people*, so naturally they bring their own opinions to the process. A child who is diagnosed with Autism by one person may be told it's PDD-NOS (that is, somethings wrong, but we just don't know what!) by someone else. In reading what symptoms all these children were experiencing, I am hoping that many of you will have those "Aha!" moments where you recognize something that you thought no other kid in the world does is actually a lot more common than you think.

Over and over I hear parents tell me their child is doing something that they write off as just a "childhood thing," "a phase," or more often as simply "weird," is actually symptomatic of a present manganese overload. The most common is nightmares. Sure, everybody has a nightmare from time to time, even a bad one, but no one should be experiencing so many that he or she becomes afraid to sleep or afraid of the dark. Many people who have told me that their child has terrible sleep issues have found out that the child was actually just afraid to go to bed! Sleep is not the bridge over troubled waters that it is to most people when you're terrified of what images your overloaded brain is going to dredge up in your sleep. Unusual fears, phobias, habits, making themselves throw up food they don't want… the list goes on and on.

For some reason some people have noted in the past that some of the people whose children saw dramatic results did not stay in touch with me after successfully completing the Protocol. There are many reasons for this and when you think about it, it's really not so strange. Why would you expect them to? Think about it; if you go to a doctor for let's say, a sore throat, do you call them later and tell them that you're feeling better? No, because you know that was what that doctor expected to happen, so you just go on with your life. It's the exact same dynamic here. They know that they had my expected result, so off they go.

It has long been my habit to write down in quotes in their charts exactly what someone has said. This has come in handy over the years as people often forget things that were going on at any given time. While it isn't always good to dwell on the past, I have, as a doctor, had to remind some of them how very far they have come by using their own words. I had a child who was on the Protocol for several months and his very stressed mom said she felt that he hadn't changed enough "despite all this cooking." I asked, "So he's still having daily tantrums and melt-downs?" Pause. "Did he used to do that?" she asked, bewildered. Yep. He sure did. I'm glad it took my notes to remind her of that and not the kid himself; he was behaving so well that apparently she kind of forgot he was once a terror! So if you see something like, "We're having so much fun now" in the narrative, that's because it was exactly what was said to me.

You will notice that the case studies all have a child's name on them, but the names are blacked out on the paperwork you will see scattered between the stories. Although I am always willing to go the extra mile to protect my clients' privacy, it felt too sterile to not refer to the kids by at least some name when I was writing the case studies. It's funny; some of them go as far back as 2005 but I could see each and every one of their faces, hear their voices, remember the funny things they said or did while I was putting these together. I even had to have the editor give them the new names because each one of them is so emblazoned on my memory I couldn't come up with any name for them except their own! Just be assured that with the exception of the names, every part of the case studies are real.

Some of these cases are long and others are short. This is simply because every case is unique! Different people respond differently. *Just remember that the reason that they had the outcomes they did is because they complied with the diet, and they hung in there.* You have to do both.

So now it's time to start your new journey. Armed with the information and the true case studies we've provided here, you'll feel good to go! It's your turn to experience the miracles of the Spectrum Balance® Protocol for yourself.

1 - 5

Even though Jay's case resolved with what seemed to be lightening speed - going from an Autism diagnosis to "not autistic" in less than three months - I had no idea if that would ever be the case again. Did we just "get lucky" with him, or could we pull off this virtual miracle again?

As it turns out, we weren't "lucky" as we would see this same pattern repeat itself over and over through the years. Although it doesn't happen this way in every case, I have seen numerous incidences of what I think of as my "Insta-kids"; cases that resolved so quickly it defied either logic or hope.

The following cases are just a few examples:

CASE STUDY 1

Mom: *"Within three days the lights came on"*

Name: Garth M. (Male)

Age: 4.5
DX: Autism
Other diets: Gluten free, FOD MAPS
RX: Nyastatin, Motrin, Benadryl
Supplements: Lotrimin Isolate, Serene, 5 HTP, TravaCor, Probiotics, Magnesium, GABA, Fish oil, Zinc, Iron, Citramins

Garth was an interesting case for many reasons. He is a perfect example of the detrimental nature of the "Band-Aid" approach to healing rather than seeking, finding and addressing the source of the issue. His many doctors had stated that he was "always low in iron" and gave him supplements, but never explored the pivotal question of *why* he was always low in iron. This case demonstrates the dramatic results that can be achieved by the Spectrum Balance Protocol because it asks (and answers) that one simple question: Why?

Garth was developing normally until he was eighteen months old, but within a month of his latest round of vaccines "he started to go down," as his mother explained. He lost all of his speech and started to have unexplained outbreaks of violence. Predictably, he was diagnosed with autism shortly thereafter. By the time I met him, he still had no speech at all (not even babbling), was not potty trained, and alarmingly, he was losing a lot of weight! He had lost eight pounds off his already sparse forty-pound frame in less than a year. As a result of this, he was quite weak and very fearful of doing anything physical.

This physical lack of confidence had unfortunately spread to all phases of his life. Garth was spending most of his time hiding out in the house, living in fear of noise, getting hurt, and even other children. Not much of a life for a four-year-old.

For many people, the diagnosis of autism constitutes an ending and incurs tremendous fear as well as a host of intense emotions. The end of thinking that your child or even your family will ever have a "normal" life. The end of your goals of taking the whole family on trips and vacations. The end of the dreams of having grandchildren. With the generally accepted pronouncement of "no known cause, no known treatment, and no known cure," for many it is the end of hope. In Garth's case, it was only the beginning of his parents' search to find something to help him that would last for the next three years.

The statement, "We've done everything," means different things to different people, but in this case I had to agree. Garth's parents really had tried everything! Immediately after his diagnosis, they had started seeing an autism specialist called a "DAN" doctor. This is a classification of medical doctor who approaches autism from both a medical and biomedical approach. The doctor had subjected Garth to extensive rounds of testing for vitamin and mineral deficiencies, heavy metals, and other toxicities. The child had been put on a series of diets and supplements meant to correct these imbalances, yet despite nearly three years of this, they had seen very little positive change in him.

Undeterred (and blessedly open-minded), the parents then tried some therapies that were outside the norm. They tried fungal detoxes, muscle testing, bio-feedback, and even traveled to Arizona for treatments designed to allow his nervous system to balance and relax. In their literature these non-invasive treatments use "frequency, vibration, sound and light" to enable a person to reach a natural state of relaxation, thereby allowing the body the ability to heal itself. Please understand that I am not saying that these treatments don't work for some people and for certain health issues; they just didn't work for Garth.

Another thing that wasn't working for Garth was his massive amount of drugs and supplements. One of his supplements alone was delivering 6 mg of manganese a day! Being that the daily recommended dosage for an adult is 2mg, this was a massive overdose for someone who only weighed forty pounds! As a traditional naturopath, I could not make any suggestions as to his prescription drugs, but I could advise about his supplements. My advice to his parents at the time was to stop giving him all of the supplements except the fish oil and probiotic.

Saying that this idea didn't sit well with his mom would be an understatement. I can't say as I blame her, since over the years she had become conditioned to the idea that he "needed" all of them and was thus fearful of stopping. Even after I explained to her how the phytate in Garth's diet was stripping him of the minerals he needed, and that eliminating phytate would allow his body to absorb the minerals from his food, she remained skeptical. So I asked her two simple questions:

"Taking all these supplements, is Garth where you want him to be?" I have often asked this question and nearly every time it appears that it is the first time anyone has ever asked parents such a direct question. The answer of course was, "Obviously not, since we're here in your office."

The second is a little TMI, but does cut right to the point. "What color is his urine?" Again, I'm good at asking questions no one has ever heard! Mom thought about it for a moment, and I could see the light come on in her head. "It's neon yellow. I guess I can figure out where his vitamins went." Yep. That one's a no-brainer... A chiropractor friend of mine actually uses that description when I ask him what he thinks of many of the new and cool supplements that seem to be launched daily. He reads the bottle and gives his pronouncement: "expensive urine." Kind of gross, but true.

After trying a multitude of diets, programs, treatments and supplements for Garth, his Mom felt that the Protocol would be an easy change. She agreed that she would start on Phase 1 of the Protocol, and despite her reservations, she would also take him off the extensive list of supplements he was currently taking. I could tell she still had reservations, but she was ready to try something new. Since they live on the West Coast, we agreed to have a phone consultation one month later.

Two-week phone call:

With most families, the hardest part of the process for them is to be able to get their mind around the specifics of the Protocol itself; what to eat, recipe suggestions, is the child consuming enough calories, etc. In Garth's case, the Protocol was actually the easy part since they had previously tried so many other far more complicated diets. The difficulty this time was to get his Mom to stop ceaselessly searching for the "next thing" to help!

The basis of this brief phone call was that she had taken her son to a nearby new practitioner who muscle tested him and said he was "high in fungus and low on calcium and magnesium." I try very hard not to disparage any other practitioners, and didn't do so here, but I again asked her a common-sense question. "Do you think Garth could be high in fungus when he's been on anti-fungals for several years?" After thinking about it, she agreed that it seemed highly unlikely and was even a tad embarrassed about it. After asking a few questions about her son's diet, it also seemed clear that he was getting plenty of calcium and magnesium from his food.

At this point I suggested what I have repeated religiously since starting my work with the Protocol -- let's look at the need for additional supplements or changes to the Protocol based on Garth's behavior rather than any additional lab or muscle testing. Again, this seems so logical but it is a concept that is not usually applied.

As for Garth himself, he was doing great! A discussion between Mom and Dad regarding how long they would stay with the Protocol without seeing any results became irrelevant when "Within three days the lights came on," as his Mom happily described. This was a little shocking to them as they had spent years doing dietary programs like gluten free and FOD MAPS only to experience negligible results, but they were thrilled with it and doubled down on being as perfect as they could with the Phase 1 foods.

Starting from that third day, Garth had maintained steady and promising progress. The habit that he had of always walking on his tiptoes had suddenly stopped from one day to the next. His mom was particularly happy as it seemed to her that his "awareness and connection seemed much higher." His nearly constant babbling that had started very early on the Protocol was already starting to take on tone and inflection, and he was listening and following directions better. His confidence was quickly growing and he was "doing physical things at the park he could never do before."

Armed with these terrific results, all in fewer than fourteen days, I gave his mom a "homework assignment" for the remainder of the month. Stay off the internet! Laughing, she replied, "Ooh. That's going to be a hard one. You're mean!"

So I'm told.

One-month progress report (phone):

"I'm very excited!" Garth's mom gushed over the phone as soon as I picked it up to greet her.

The rapid progress that he had made in the first two weeks was not showing any signs of slowing down. The improved cognitive ability and acuity that she had mentioned before was continuing unabated. He was now actively working on talking, and was quick to learn by association -- that is, putting food in the bowl, bubbles in the bath, etc. His babbling was all "happy sounding talk" and he was trying out singing.

Garth's growing confidence was showing itself in improved eye contact (even with people he didn't know well), and he had begun climbing and jumping when he was at the park -- something he couldn't accomplish either physically or emotionally before. His mind and his body were becoming stronger, and he was emerging from his world of fears and turning into a happy boy.

The one hang up was in his potty training. When I asked about that, his mother told me, "He knows what I want him to do and how to do it. He's being purposely stubborn."   While I'm sure it was a pain for his mom, being stubborn is a choice and at least he was making choices, which I saw as progress. Easy for me to say, right?

As for the Protocol, his mom admitted that they had probably been eating too much off the "moderate" food list, but by using my own yardstick, it was hard to argue with the results Garth was exhibiting. As Garth was becoming more aware, he was also getting more picky about his food instead of just eating whatever she put in front of him, and he was wanting more of the "moderate" foods. I suggested that Mom continue on making sure he was eating as many of the "best" choice foods as she could, but to keep him eating. It was obviously working!

Two-month progress report: (phone)

This month's conversation held some wonderful news. Garth's grandmother, a registered nurse, had pronounced that he was "no longer autistic" as he was not exhibiting any of the symptoms that were needed for that diagnosis! Obviously, there were areas where he needed to catch up, but it was also obvious that he was going to do it, and do it quickly.

His newfound confidence was "going through the roof," as his mother described. She laughed, "I could put him on the phone with you. He wants to do everything himself." Thankfully, this included his bathroom behavior, as he had decided to potty train himself.

In the short time of this past month, his speech had transformed itself from happy babbling to words, then to little phrases, and then into more conceptual speech. For example, his mom told me that she told Garth, "Say goodbye to Daddy" and he replied, "I already did."

Garth had transformed from being a silent, scared little boy to a happy, confident and chatty kid in fewer than sixty days. After years of

trying everything they could find his family was completely aston-
ished that such a small change in diet from what they had been doing
had created such a monumental change. They were now seeing a
Garth emerging who they never had guessed existed. "He's so hilar-
ious and so smart," his mom reported. "We went to a BBQ and he
went over and said hello to everyone."

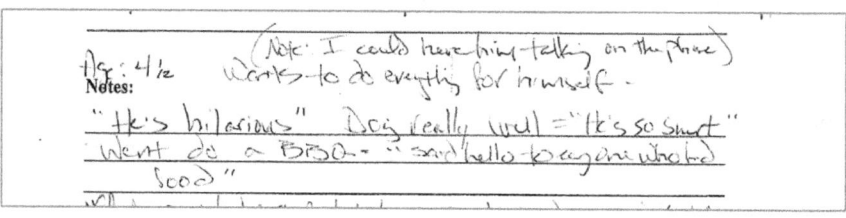

Most times at this point where there is so much improvement, I suggest that they start moving from Phase 2 of the diet to Phase 3, which
is a slightly modified regular Paleo diet. This time I decided I wanted to keep him on Phase 2 a bit longer, mostly because he had previously been taking the aforementioned high-manganese supplement
for years. Ever watch a fireman putting out a match on the ground?
He keeps grinding it until he's positive it's out. You could say I'm
like that with manganese!

Three-month progress report: (phone)

Garth's progress was shooting through the roof now. "He's on fire"
were the words his exalted mom used to describe his progress to me.
"He's happy, super confidant, and is playing with other kids."

Now that he was speaking so much, they had noticed a possible
slight apraxia and had hired a speech therapist. When I spoke to him
on the phone, he sounded age appropriate to me, but then again, I
don't speak to him every day. Since working with his new therapist
he still had "lots and lots of baby talk" and was doing well in putting

sentences together. They had some work to do but he was rapidly catching up.

During this phone call, an interesting nugget was revealed: Garth's mom told me that she had been working for years with a chapter of a famous autism group (that is also sponsored by a famous female celebrity). She had told the nutritionist for the group about the amazing and nearly instant progress her son had made and had given her a copy of the Protocol. The nutritionist at the time, according to Mom, said that she was "fascinated" and would get in immediate touch with me. Apparently this conversation had occurred months ago, so I guess her idea of immediately is different from mine. Garth's mom was very surprised that the nutritionist had not gotten in touch with me, and said that she would talk to her again. This happened back in 2009, and as of this writing, still "radio silence."

As surprised as Garth's mom was, I was not surprised at all as this was just one of many doctors, specialists, and autism groups that had promised parents they would call me immediately yet I would never hear from them. I had been working with the Protocol for almost four years at this point and had gotten used to them not burning up my phone lines.

Suddenly during this pivotal phone call, I had (what I thought) was a brilliant idea. Since this nutritionist was so highly placed in such a famous and well-funded autism group, what if Mom took Garth in to be re-evaluated by this woman herself? Then this nutritionist could actually see with her own eyes what we had been able to accomplish with Garth in such a short period of time. Perhaps if she saw the proof of the Protocol's impact, then it could take us a giant step forward in getting the Protocol the attention it deserves in the autism world! Great idea, right?

Well…not so much. When I brought this idea up to Mom, it was obvious that I had stepped on a nerve. I had no idea why it received such a chilly reception, so I asked if there was a problem. As it turned out, the predominant number of doctors, treatments, and specialists Garth had seen -- including his current speech therapist -- were all paid for by government programs for special needs kids. If he wasn't "autistic," then that funding would cease. Then I made a critical error. As excited as I was at the prospect of such a large and media-friendly autism organization spreading the word that some hope for these kids was found, I pressed her. I asked: "What do you think is more important -- the extra funds from the programs Garth actually no longer needs, or the idea that so many more kids could be helped, like your son was, by this Protocol?" She said she'd think about it. The conversation lasted a few more uncomfortable minutes, then mercifully ended.

<u>Follow up:</u>

To be truthful, I'm not exactly sure of what happened next. I don't know what all her thought process entailed, but I never heard from her again, and my phone calls to her went unanswered. She may very well have tried (and failed) with the nutritionist and her organization, but I guess I'll never know for sure. I do know that this was not the first and far from the last time I ran up against the government or state aid situation, even alimony a few times, and that when it comes to finances things can get very tricky. I suppose I shouldn't be too surprised since we all know the expression, money talks, right? Fortunately now, so does Garth!

CASE STUDY 2

Mom: *"It's so exciting. He's just a typical two-and-a-half-year-old boy."*

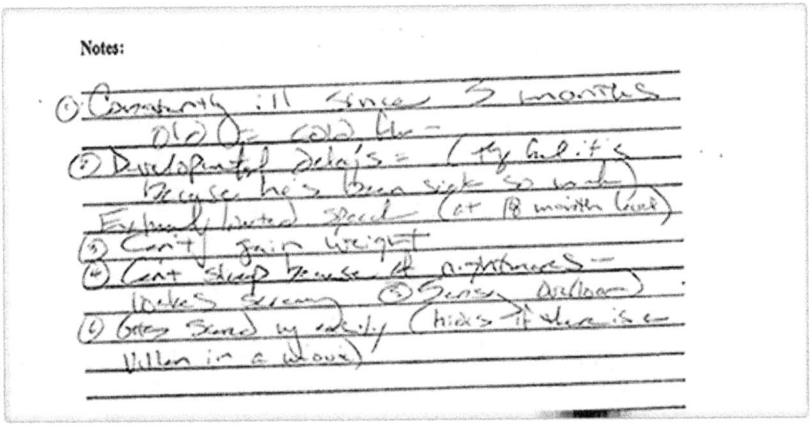
Notes:

① Constantly ill since 3 months old [illegible] – cold, flu –

② Developmental delays = (they feel it's because he's been sick so much) Extremely limited speech (at 18 months [illegible])

③ Can't gain weight

④ Can't sleep because of nightmares – wakes screaming ⑤ Sensory overload

⑥ Gets scared very easily (hides if there is a villain in a movie)

Name: Paxton G. (Male)

Age: 2.5
DX: None officially
Other diets: Clean and organic, but lots of grains

You'll notice throughout the book that I mention how much I love working with the really little kids like this. I know I repeat this often, but it's hard to express how much fun it is because they change so quickly. It's like watching one of those time-lapse films where you see a rose blooming from a bud to a flower in just a few minutes. And there is nothing that can compare with watching kids bloom!

Over the years I've seen the attitudes of the parents vary wildly; everything from intense disbelief and resistance, to being hungry for knowledge and ready for anything. Paxton's mom was one who came in raring to go and ready to do everything I suggested. This is not only easier on me, but it makes better use of the time I have for them to discuss food options and the like instead of spending extra time on the science behind the Protocol.

Although not diagnosed (on purpose) there was a lot "not right" with Paxton and his mom was eager to get to the bottom of it.

By the time I saw him he was only two-and-a-half years old, and the poor guy had already experienced multiple health issues. Since he was three months old he'd been "sick constantly." Colds, flu, anything that was going around, he got it, and as a result had very low energy. Paxton also had a lot of developmental delays, but his parents were having a hard time figuring out if that was because he was sick all the time or if there were other issues. Other than the constant illnesses, he had developed pretty normally up until about eighteen months and then stopped in his tracks; now, at almost three he was still at that eighteen-month-old level. That was enough of a concern that there were other issues at work for them to bring him to see me. The whole story sounded an alarm bell for me.

As if being sniffly all the time wasn't bad enough on such a little guy, he had some very sad and inexplicable emotional problems. His sensory overload issues were making mountains out of molehills in every area of his life. Not only did light hurt his eyes and every little sound drive him crazy, this overload was also crossing over into his emotional life. Mom described him as "afraid of everything" to the point that if there was any kind of a bad guy in a TV show he would hide, usually under furniture. He was terrified of even the smallest dog, or of someone coming to the door of the house. Worst of all, he was waking screaming from nightmares several times a week. This was made even harder since he would not allow any level of affection because he hated being touched. As you can imagine, this was devastating to his loving parents who couldn't even comfort their own crying child.

When you hear the phrase "sensory overload" it conjures the image of light and sound sensitivity, and that is the main symptom of it. What is often overlooked is the emotional aspect of it -- fear. For many of these children, they feel that people like siblings, teachers, kids at school, even their parents "hate them." Because their sensitivity to light and sound are so high, they tend to have a perception that everyone is yelling at them. Imagine if you went to work and everyone there yelled at you all day, every day. You'd start thinking everybody hated you pretty quickly too. This is very often why these kids become "defiant" or "mean." In their minds they're not doing anything wrong, they're just defending themselves. In this case though, Paxton was far away from being described as "mean." He just stayed scared.

Mom and I went over Phase 1 of the Protocol, which she assured me every member of the family (including the new baby on her lap) would be starting that very day. She was very interested in being able to strictly adhere to Phase 1, and said five of my favorite words before leaving: "I'm so excited about this." In my experience, that attitude virtually guarantees success.

One-month progress report:

Between his young age and his mom's enthusiasm for the Protocol, it was not a surprise to me that Paxton was doing so well. You know you've come to a strange point in your career when these miraculous changes that occur on the Protocol start to become part of an average Tuesday! After seeing this happen with so many children, the "miracles" the families report have had a tendency to become more like "expected results" to me. Wonderful, but expected.

Mom, however, was over the moon at all the new changes. As is the norm with these little ones, there were exciting new things happening daily. There was a lot to report about his sensory and emotional issues, and I was very glad to hear that he had not been sick. This was the longest he had ever gone without getting something since he was three months old. He seemed more robust as well and had gained an entire size in his baby clothes. Best of all, his mom reported that he now had "amazing energy."

His speech, which had been stunted at eighteen months, suddenly soared. His speech therapist said his progress this month was "huge." He was not only gaining new words on a daily basis, but he was much more intelligible, and putting words and concepts together for himself.

With all his exciting gains, Paxton had some wonderful losses as well. The nightmares that had woken him screaming several times a week had suddenly ceased after just a few days on the Protocol. Gone too was his extreme sensitivities to light and sound, and with his world seeming calmer, he was too.

When I asked about the "afraid of everything" situation, Mom had to think for a bit. "It's a lot different. He's sensitive to things but I think that's just who he is." Very wise. No two people are alike and I love to see a parent who is letting their kids be themselves, instead of who they think they should be. Paxton was having no problems with regular TV shows now, he just didn't really like the darker ones. No problems with little dogs, just cautious with the big ones. He had turned from acting out of fear, to making his own choices.

There was no hesitation from Mom when I asked what her favorite change was in the last thirty days. After about a week on the Protocol when his parents were putting him to bed, Paxton asked if they would lay down with him for awhile. This had never happened before. "For the first time in his life we can cuddle with him. He asks for us to lay down at night with him now. He would never cuddle and now he loves it." Maybe a therapist would have picked something else out as the best or biggest change that took place in that month, but not a mother. Moms will always take the cuddling.

Paxton's new lack of fear and distaste for affection were even boldly displayed to me. As they were getting ready to leave, he asked if he could look to see what was on my computer screen. When I said yes, he walked over and casually climbed up on my lap as if he'd been there a hundred times, hanging his arm around my neck. After asking his questions, he said, "Thank you, gotta go!" gave me a hug and went back to his mom. Obviously, big changes in the little man.

Two-month progress report:

"It's so exciting. He's just a typical two-and-a-half-year-old boy."

Yep. That about summed it up. After only sixty days on the Protocol, Paxton had become a typical boy his age. Physically, he looked hardy and strong with a much improved muscle tone than he had started with. I'm sure it helped that he hadn't been sick at all, and he was now at an appropriate weight and height for his age. His speech was rapidly and constantly improving, and was much more coherent and conversational. While walking upstairs to my office for his appointment, he held my hand and excitedly told me all about a picnic his family had been on recently.

Thankfully, the sensory overload was gone and had taken all its frightening and nasty symptoms along with it. Although he did have one bad dream that month, it was a far cry from the screaming nightmares he used to experience several times a week. His mom was actually impressed that when he woke from it he came all the way down the dark hallway by himself to ask if he could get in bed with them, something he would have never attempted in his former terrified state.

Paxton's desire for affection was continuing to blossom and was now branching out beyond the immediate family. At a recent gathering he was very comfortable and happy playing with the other kids, and even gave an affectionate hug to comfort a crying cousin. Not only was he now affectionate, he was also becoming compassionate. Growing up…

As there were no negative symptoms left to work on, I discharged Paxton in August of 2013 on a standard Paleo diet, which his whole family follows.

Follow up:

I see Paxton often when he comes in with his mom to pick up supplements in the office. He always graces me with a wave and an exuberant greeting, "Hi, Dr. Shauna!" accompanied by a big hug. He is very social and polite and always makes it a point to say hello to all the staff, but he makes me feel special. I'm the only one he singles out to hold hands with and to tell his stories whenever I have time to talk. His vocabulary is impressive and he is a pretty competent storyteller; he's also just such a sweet boy. It's funny. His family was hoping that he could become "typical" and instead they got "extraordinary." I don't think they mind.

CASE STUDY 3

Notes (handwritten):
- look Prefull's — (Did he's ADDness)
- Age: 1 (on formula) = has been on formula = ready for pureed food
- Always been a tough baby — fussy, colicky, my old reactive to "earthy" "He came out crazy"
- Very first mood swings = "zero to 100 in half a heartbeat"
- Terribly sensitive to noise = Plush

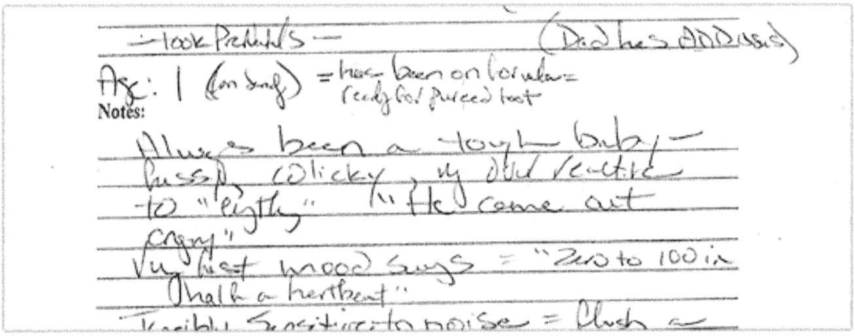

Name: Kyle P. (Male)

Age: 1 year
DX: None officially
Other diets: Baby formula

As healthcare providers it if often thought that we shouldn't have favorites. But hey, we're all human! So, I'll just go ahead and admit that this little guy was one of my all-time favorites. Working with little babies like this is so incredible because they change on a nearly daily basis. Although I like working with all the kids, the under-two-year-olds are the most...I guess you'd say...fun! It's amazing how much change can happen in such a small amount of time when the protocol is adhered to completely and they have no bad habits to overcome like adults do. Babies rarely stop for fast food on their way home from work.

In many cases the families and I have to do quite a bit of detective work to ascertain where the source of the excess manganese might be, but in this case it was pretty much of a slam dunk. Not only was he on baby formula that had very high concentrations of manganese; his mother had taken a prenatal vitamin that had 4 mg of it in it as well. Case closed.

The first words out of his mom's mouth were, "He came out angry." Even though she had had an uneventful pregnancy that made them feel that there would be nothing to worry about, Kyle just didn't act like other babies. There was no cuddling or touching to the point that he wouldn't even breastfeed. Of all the possible symptoms, I think that this is one of the most heartbreaking of all of them. As a parent you wait nine long months dreaming about holding and cuddling your precious newborn, only to have your baby reject you. Sometimes for years.

There were any number of things that seemed off kilter about Kyle. He had an extreme sensitivity to noise, and was described as "over reactive to everything." He had awful mood swings, which his mom described as "zero to one hundred in half a heartbeat." He was constantly flapping and stimming, which made keeping him under control during the appointment a rather interesting exercise. He was such a cute little muffin who was made a whole lot less cute by screaming at the top of his lungs and hitting at anyone who came near him the whole time, including his mother. It wasn't the first time (or the last) I was grateful that my office is upstairs from the waiting room and has a door that closes.

A little after his first birthday passed, Kyle still had zero speech, not even baby babbling, and Mom finally faced the idea that something might be wrong with her child. Always a bad day for any parent. She also could not figure out why he always seemed tired. Why would a one-year-old who does not even walk yet be so exhausted? I wondered if he was experiencing poor sleep from the bad dreams that are so common with Menefe Syndrome, but since he couldn't talk I couldn't ask him.

Since Kyle was only a year old, there was a challenge as to how to get the Protocol foods into him, as the bulk of his diet thus far had been formula. Going through the list of the most beneficial foods, his mom and I came up with some recipes that she felt she could puree for him and that he would eat. She was ready to start.

One-month progress report:

I love good news, and Mom had great news for me. She was amazed that many noticeable changes had started taking place almost instantly when they took him off the formula he had been eating. His progress was extremely swift and as she put it he "mellowed out in two weeks."

The mood swings and anger were gone, and he was much more easy going. He was even developing an unexpected sense of humor! His energy was way up and overall he appeared to be much happier. Although not exactly cuddly he was no longer pushing people away or hitting. He even let me hold him this time (no way on the first visit) and made excellent eye contact with me while sitting on my lap. He was much calmer, with the flapping and stimming gone with no reappearance after the very first week. He had stopped lining up toys (a symptom often looked for in an Autism diagnosis) and started playing with them instead, sometimes entertaining himself for long periods. As Mom said: "He's enjoying himself and figuring things out for himself." In other words, acting age-appropriate. Excellent.

After the first week on the protocol Kyle started to babble on a regular basis and even pulled his very first word, "Dada," out of his bag of new tricks. A few days after that eventful word, he spontaneously pulled himself up on the coffee table and casually walked over to his father, who was sitting open-mouthed on the couch. Smart kid. Dada up to that point had been a bit of a skeptic and not really on board with the Protocol, but after being featured as his first word coupled with Kyle's stroll across the living room, he was now an enthusiastic supporter.

There were no negatives to report, and since they were fully on board about sticking with the Protocol, I discharged Kyle from seeing me monthly.

Follow up:

After only one month, a cute little blond-haired, blue eyed baby boy had taken the place of the once angry, screaming child. Kyle was discharged in July 2010 and never looked back.

CASE STUDY 4

Mom: *"I was afraid I'd have to institutionalize him. It's good to know it's diet!"*

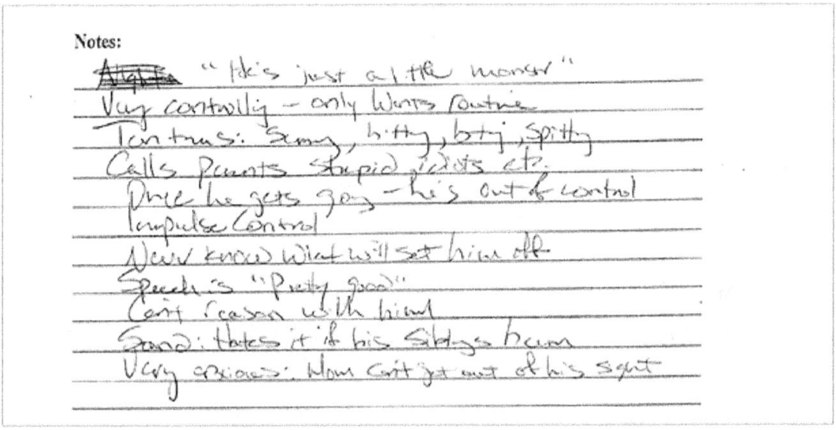

Notes:

[handwritten notes, partially legible:]

"He's just a little monster"

Very controlling – only wants routine

Tantrums: screamy, hitting, biting, spitting

Calls parents stupid idiots etc.

Once he gets going – he's out of control

Impulse control

Never know what will set him off

Speech is "pretty good"

Can't reason with him

Sound: hates it if his siblings hum

Very anxious: Mom can't get out of his sight

Name: Dennis W. (Male)

Age: 6
DX: None officially but all his programs were geared toward autism
ND: Linda Kane
Other diets: Orphanage food, baby formula. Clean whole food after adoption.

Dennis was one of many referrals from a wonderful neurodevelopmentalist I have worked with for many years named Linda Kane (her real name used with permission). Linda and her group, "A Hope and a Future," have done so much incredible work for children with various neurological issues over the years it was inevitable that we would find each other. Combining our Protocols has created some amazing outcomes and the woman is truly an angel.

One of the reasons I am including Dennis in these case studies is because this was done completely on the phone. It is very important to note that this Protocol can be done by parents at home and still provide terrific outcomes, as people have seen in the sixty-seven countries where it is currently downloaded.

With as rough a start as Dennis got in life, it was easy to blame his behavioral issues on the trauma he endured already in his young life. Even though he was just shy of two years old when he was adopted, life in a Guatemalan orphanage could not have been easy, especially for a child with visual disabilities. Children as we know, can be cruel. After his adoption, his wonderful new parents put him immediately on whole, fresh, and organic foods, but the awful orphanage meals had already taken their toll.

Many people I've worked with fall into the "we've tried everything" category, and Dennis' parents certainly qualified. The ND work had helped his vision enormously but had not been as effective for his behavioral problems as they would like to have seen. They tried a program using sequential homeopathics for over two years (at $500 a month) that had yielded little -- Dennis had gained a little bit of speech and had stopped drooling. They had tried "every diet on the planet," said his mother, every "treatment" that promised hope -- all to no avail. And yet here they were, still willing to try something new. After four years of trying everything, they still had hope.

Phone consultations pose a whole new set of challenges for me, and I had to find the right method to obtain as much of the information I needed as possible. What I wound up doing was asking what questions I could ask the parent in order to know that a child is improving, and then asked those same questions each time we spoke. That turned out to be incredibly helpful, especially since people sometimes have short memories. Since I never met Dennis, the case study description will sound a bit more clinical and less personal than the ones that came into the office.

When I asked my first question about his overall state, and what she wanted to work on, Mom heaved a big sigh. I've heard a lot of these "where do I begin" sighs, so I waited for her to gather her thoughts. After a pause she said, "Well...he's just a little monster."

It was hard to know where to begin with Dennis because of his overall extreme behavior. Screaming, hitting, biting, and spitting were all a constant reaction from him. He was very controlling and if absolutely everything did not go his way and according to his routine then the parents were in for a massive melt-down. The boy's description for nearly everyone was to call them "a stupid idiot" or to become physically abusive. He had no impulse control and no apparent trigger that the family could avoid. "We never know what's going to set him off and once he gets going there is no reasoning with him. He just spins out of control," his mother described.

Added to all of this alarming physical behavior was the fact that he had to have his mother in his direct sight at all times. If he could not see her he became extremely anxious and agitated, and would spin even further out of control. While his behavior was a burden on the entire family, this trait made it even more torturous for his mother, who could never have a moment away from him.

Although I start everyone out on Phase 1 of the Protocol we decided that because his symptoms were so acute, we would take it one step further. I suggested that she give him foods from only the "best" choice food list to see if we could kick start his progress. Based on the strong referral to me from his ND, his exhausted mom was willing to try anything. Fortunately since the family was already eating organic whole foods, the change was not as difficult as it is for many.

One-month progress report: (phone)

In stark contrast from our first conversation where I would have described her as cautiously hopeful, Dennis' mom was on fire! Bub-

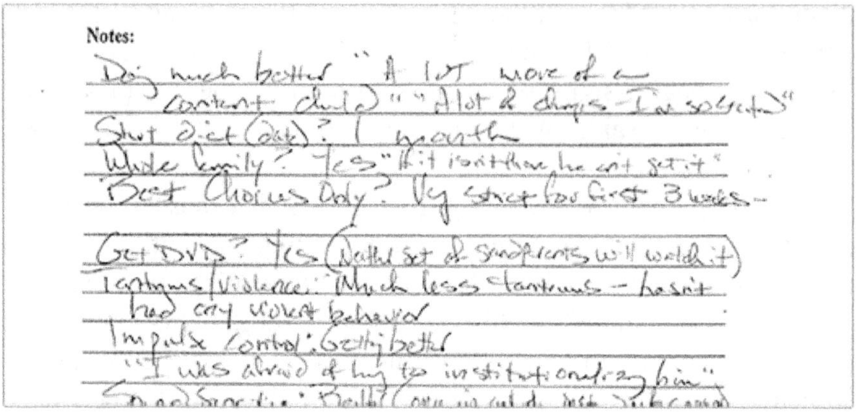

Notes:

[handwritten notes, partially legible:]
Doing much better "A lot more of a content child." "Alot of changes - I'm so excited."
Shut diet (daily)? 1 month
Whole family? Yes "if it isn't there he cant get it."
Best Choices Only? Very strict for first 3 weeks -

Get DVD? Yes (Nutri set of supplements will watch it)
tantrums/violence: Much less tantrums - he isn't had any violent behavior
Impulse control: both better
"I was afraid of having to institutionalize him"

bling with enthusiasm she was talking faster than I could write today. When I asked how it was going, she responded, "There are so many changes! I'm so excited!" Some of my favorite words…

Even though I had told her during our initial phone call that she could expect to see some changes in her son fairly quickly, I have learned over time that it is one thing to hear it, and a far different thing to actually witness it for yourself. After putting the whole family on the Protocol as I suggested she started to see positive changes in Dennis almost immediately. In a steady day-to-day progression, she watched her son transforming before her eyes. He became much calmer and less controlling, and as hard as his behavior had been on the whole family, his mom had been more concerned about the toll it was taking on her son. Her relief was evident when she said, "He's a much more content child."

The multiple daily tantrums and name calling were melting away, and his physical violence had completely abated, Mom reported. His impulse control was steadily improving and she was noticing that she could actually reason with him; something that was impossible before.

About two weeks into the Protocol, she was working in the kitchen and suddenly noticed that Dennis wasn't there. Since he had such extreme separation anxiety and had to be able to physically see her at all times, she immediately became concerned that something had happened to him. After a frantic search around the house, she found him sitting on the floor in his room, playing quietly with some toys.

The family was having no trouble at all adhering to the Protocol, and were having some very pleasant "side effects." Both she and her husband were losing weight, and her own anxiety, which she had not mentioned before, was quelled. Although I felt sure that most of that was because Dennis was doing so much better, she said she also felt that part of it was attributed to the Protocol. She was using some of the many Paleo recipe sites to give her ideas, and they were easily finding new family favorites to enjoy.

"It's good to know that it's diet - I can control that. I was afraid it was the adoption thing."

Two-month progress report: (phone)

One of the biggest roadblocks with this Protocol, is that even when the child, and his or her parents and siblings are all on board, you still have the most common saboteur to deal with: the grandparents. While visiting with relatives, Dennis' grandparents arbitrarily decided that "a little won't hurt him" and against the directives of his parents, they were sneaking him cookies when Mom and Dad were out of the room. A lot of older children on the Protocol will actually argue with their grandparents when this happens, and I've heard of some pretty epic lectures from the kids about staying on "their program," but Dennis was six. Kind of hard for a six-year-old to resist cookies!

The result was nearly immediate. Although Dennis did not revert to his former state of constant melt-downs and tantrums, the verbal abuse came roaring back, and once again, everyone was a "stupid head." A big, old screaming tantrum brought it to his parents attention that something was definitely amiss, and out came the cookie confession.

Now that his parents identified the source of the problem, they put him back very strictly on Phase 1 for a week. "It was so amazing," his mom said. "He came right back." Moving him back to Phase 2 after that week went very smoothly too and with no negative effects. Whew! Dennis was back.

Since the child had no issues as long as he was on the Protocol, we let his next phone appointment go a few months while staying on Phase 2 to see how things went. We set up our next phone appointment for just after Thanksgiving. The holidays are often tricky, but after the cookie monster episode, Mom felt the rest of the extended family would be more likely to be on board!

Five-month progress report: (phone)

Despite the fact that they had not been "extremely strict" over the holidays, Dennis sailed through like a champ. Originally described as a "little monster" the family now enjoyed a tamer, happier "regular six-year-old." Content, bright, and growing like a weed, Dennis was now calm and reasonable. The violence and melt-downs were quickly becoming just a bad memory, and his anxiety was non-existent. Although he still enjoyed hanging out with Mom, he had no problem when she wasn't there.

After all their years of searching for something to "help" Dennis, his parents found instead that he had virtually changed into a different child. In only five months their expectations had changed from "I don't want to have to institutionalize him" to "I have great hopes for him now." Dennis had some catching up to do, but he had a great team behind him to help.

When I am getting ready to discharge a client, I always have one of my many versions of "the talk" with them, since it is vital that people understand that they can not go back to their old SAD way of eating. With this family it was virtually unnecessary since they were all whole food eaters anyway. When I told his mom she could go to Phase 3, but I suggest they stay there, she commented, "There is such a difference in all the kids, not just Dennis. This is the way we eat now."

Follow up:

I discharged Dennis on Phase 3, December of 2011. I told Mom to call if there were any issues in the future, and I suggested they stay with their ND work until Dennis had fully caught up. Not surprisingly, that call never came.

CASE STUDY 5

Name: Mason R. (Male)

Age: 3
DX: PDD-NOS
Other diets: Soy baby formula

The main reason that I am including Mason in these case studies is because he was displaying so many symptoms that are **not** normally considered to be part of the autism spectrum that nevertheless were able to be resolved with the Protocol. Yes, he had many of the more common symptoms; enough so that the doctor who diagnosed him with PDD-NOS said that he would most likely "become autistic," but for now, he was "missing a few symptoms" for that specific diagnosis. After seeing Mason myself and comparing him with other children, I strongly believe that many other doctors would probably have given him the autism label.

While having high sensory input is extremely common, Mason had the most unusual one as his prime issue. He was very sensitive to light to the point of covering his eyes and crying from bright light, but his main area of sensitivity was touch. He literally could not stand to have anything touching his skin. Shirts, diapers, bed covers and anyone touching him all drove him crazy, and it was getting progressively worse. How is a parent supposed to deal with a three-year-old who refuses to keep his clothes on? Very frustrating and sad, too.

Mason's speech had taken a sharp nose dive, and he only spoke in very slow, garbled "sort of words." Because he had been talking well before his latest round of vaccines, his mom felt that the vaccines damaged him. The timing certainly pointed to that as a possibility, but I felt strongly that more of the problems had been caused by the high manganese in his soy baby formulas. Perhaps the vaccines were the straw that finally broke the camel's back for him.

Whenever I work with the kids I always try to get them to respond to me as much as they are capable of to get an idea of how they interact with people and the world. In Mason's case, boy I got nothing. Far from being able to make that simple eye contact, I was not entirely sure if he even knew I was in the room. He did not look up when being spoken to, and seemed to be completely in his own world. When I asked his mom if that might be because he is leery of doctors (or just people) she shook her head. "He really has no awareness of other people. He doesn't even seem to have any emotions or feelings about himself, other than to take his clothes off." I again questioned the PDD-NOS diagnosis in my mind. If this wasn't autism, what was?

During our first appointment, Mason's nearly uncontrollable hyperactivity he had shown thus far suddenly just shut down. One second he was struggling and squalling, and the next moment he was lying on the floor staring absently out the window. It was so sudden it shocked me, but as it turns out, this was very common for him. "He only has two energy levels -- hyperactive or completely worn out."

He never wanted to go outside or play even in his hyperactive states, and did not have the attention span to be read to or play games in his fatigued state. While looking at him lying motionless on the floor, Mom remarked, "It just isn't natural for a three-year-old to be so tired." I agreed!

At first his mom seemed almost offended that I wasn't one-hundred percent on board with the idea that this stemmed solely from vaccine damage. Since I am a naturopath, many seem to believe that this would be my knee jerk reaction. I explained to her that while I did not discount the idea that the vaccines had been involved, I strongly felt that it was mostly the high manganese that was causing his issues. After looking through the food lists of the Protocol, she sighed again and asked me the question that so many others would in the future. "Isn't there just a pill or a treatment or something we can do instead?"

No. There isn't. It amazes me how many people would rather take their kids to a doctor or treatment center several times a week, or daily in some cases I've seen, than to undertake a dietary change. This case took place back in 2005, a mere few months into my using the Protocol, when I still had no idea of the amount of resistance I would see to merely changing food. Even all these years later I still can't figure out a person who will take their child to a doctor to get B12 shots three or four times a week, but considers a dietary change to be "too much trouble." Seems to me it's quicker to go the grocery store once a week.

Over time my attitude with people, out of necessity, has become a bit more "take it or leave it." I give them all the information I can, resources for even more, and the ability to call and email the No Harm Foundation for advice, but then I have to let go and leave it up to them. As I've said for years, you can lead a horse to water but you can't make it take its supplements. But being that this one was only a few months in, I desperately wanted her to get Mason on it and spent the next fifteen minutes trying to persuade her by telling her about all the wonderful successes I had had thus far in using the Protocol. She eventually said she'd "give it a shot." Not quite the ringing endorsement I was hoping for, but it was obviously as good as I was going to get.

One-month follow up:

As it so often happens with the little ones like this, Mason's symptoms had begun changing for the better within the first week. I could tell right away from the big smile he was giving me as he sat swinging his legs in his chair. On the first appointment he was staring right through me. Today, he was actively interested in both me and his surroundings; especially my extensive rubber duck collection.

While it is more common to see symptoms taper off, sometimes they just *poof* and disappear, and it had happened that way with Mason. The extreme sensitivity to anything touching him had simply just stopped one night. He went to bed with it, he woke up the next day without it. One of the best parts of working with such young children is that they aren't in behavioral ruts like the rest of us, and don't have old habits to break. All Mason knew is that one day it hurt, but now it doesn't. End of story.

It was immediately obvious that his eye contact was much better, since he rarely took his eyes off me for the whole appointment, but with it was coming an enormous change in his perception of the world. "He's seeing and responding to things that he would have never even noticed before," Mom marveled. Not only was he noticing people, he was becoming friendly to them and developing a sweet sense of humor.

His speech was growing by leaps and bounds with daily improvement and "tons of new words," along with the new skill of responding to questions with his words instead of gestures. It became apparent to them that Mason was now understanding what was being said to him because he seemed to be applying the appropriate emotion along with his language. For example, his babysitter had been very upset because she had lost her cat. A few days later, when she was telling Mason's mom that the cat had come home, Mason commented, "Oh, good!" and gave the babysitter a big hug. Words, understanding, and compassion. All were very positive signs.

His hyperactive/worn out swings had quickly evened out as well. He was now asking to play outside by himself and with other kids. "He wants to walk and run and play now." He had plenty of energy but when I asked if she would characterize it as hyperactive, his mom laughed and said "No more than any other three-year-old." His quiet times were now more fun too, since he would easily settle down and play with toys or a quiet game. His new favorite things to do were having the babysitter read to him, and to work on his conversational skills by having "talks" with either his parents or the babysitter; talks he would initiate himself. His world was expanding quickly and he was ready!

When I asked his mom (as I always do) what there issues there were to work on, she really had to think about it. She looked at her son, who was smiling and calmly sitting in his chair. Finally she said, "It sounds crazy but I really can't think of anything. He needs a little more language, but that's already happening so fast."

As it turns out, the Protocol was not as difficult as she had imagined (not to mention that both she and her husband had lost weight), so my suggestion that they stick to it was met with much more enthusiasm this time. Being that I had only been working with the Protocol for a few months, it had not yet morphed into the Phase 1, 2, and 3 that it is today, and "staying on it" only consisted of two food lists. The ones that were okay to eat, and the high-manganese list to avoid. It is much more sophisticated now and with many more foods included, but at the time, even the early version had done the trick for Mason.

Since I now had a good twenty or so manganese cases under my belt, I was beginning to write a scientific paper about the phenomenon I had discovered. I asked Mason's mother, as I had asked all the moms, to write a brief journal or testimonial about Mason's rapid recovery to include with my paper. She told me that she absolutely would and would bring it in for their next month's appointment.

Follow-up:

As it would continue to happen in the future, I never heard from them again, nor did I receive that testimonial. I've found that it is very hard to get people to put the time aside to do it when the kids are doing so fantastic!

As much as I would like to know how all the kids are doing, there is one thing I have comforted myself with over the years. As a general rule, if the child starts to regress in any way shape or form (always from food by the way), then I hear from their moms and/or dads. It's usually in the form of an email telling me how badly they "messed up" with their diet and requesting the latest version of the Protocol to get "touched up" again. And when they continue to do well, occasionally, I will hear from the relative or the person who referred them to me about how "great" they are doing. I guess this is what they mean when they say "no news is good news".

CHAPTER FOUR

New Science

At this point it became clear that we needed a catchy name to describe this imbalance of manganese and iron, as no one had coined one as of yet. Since the elemental table abbreviation for manganese is MN, and iron is FE, we now began referring to this condition as the "Menefe Syndrome."

Before I go into the specifics of Menefe Syndrome and its symptoms, I think it's important to understand the enormity of the autism/ASD problem. In the 1980s the prevalence of autism was reported to be one in ten thousand. In the 1990s it was one in twenty-five hundred. The most recent estimate is now a staggering one in fifty. Many say that this is because it is now being diagnosed more, and I do believe that has some merit, but I have reason to have another opinion. **Even with one in fifty children now receiving an official diagnosis, I would estimate that more than half of the children I work with have received no such official diagnosis, and are therefore not included in this number.** So even though there are more cases being reported, maybe even some that are iffy, there is a vast number of affected children who are not included in those statistics. It begs the question: What is the "real" number?

With the statistics so high, chances are that you know someone with autism or with something considered to be on the autism spectrum; like ADD, sensory input disorder, PDD-NOS ... it seems the list expands every week. One of the things that has never ceased to amaze me is the ability so many have to completely ignore the obvious. With the horrific rise in ASDs in children and in various neurological and psychological conditions in adults in such a short amount of time, what could it possibly be besides their diet? It's the only logical explanation. Yes, we live with a terrible amount of new toxins, but doesn't everything come back to what kind of fuel is in your tank? Not all of us work in toxic environments, or live in polluted urban areas, had vaccines, or were raised on soy baby formulas. **Our only common denominator is that we all eat.**

So what is Menefe Syndrome? First of all, you will be very unlikely to see anything on Menefe Syndrome that is not directly related to me, which is something I'm working to change. It is a term I coined and as I said, it is new science.

Here is the official description: "It is a highly-disruptive and pervasive condition resulting from a dietary pattern and/or other environmental factors and exposures, either very early in life or later in life, that overloads the body burden of the element manganese while at the same time provides levels of consumed anti-nutrients such as phytic acid/ phytate that act to block bioavailability of a number of essential minerals including iron, which action can defeat otherwise naturally regulated homeostasis between manganese and iron within the body and especially within developing or adult brain tissues. This syndrome has the potential to contribute answers both for causation, remedies and prevention for a broad range of Autism Spectrum Disorders (ASDs) as well as a diverse range of other potentially related health challenging conditions that negatively impact massive and escalating numbers of children and adults worldwide."

Whew!

In other words, Menefe Syndrome is characterized by the relationship between iron and manganese in your body. Iron and manganese use the same receptor sites in your brain. They are supposed to balance one another, but when the manganese gets the upper hand it creates a pattern of recognizable symptoms. If you think of it in the simplest of terms, iron is often used to convey information, such as in its use in wiring and communication cables. Manganese stores information, like in its use in batteries. When there is too much manganese over iron, manganese overwhelms the iron in the receptor sites -- this results in extremely high sensory input because the input is stored instead of being recognized and moving on.

This can manifest in a huge variety of symptoms. I'm going to touch on the most common in children.

An enhanced or even extreme sensitivity to light. This can present itself in symptoms such as not wanting to go outside, always wanting their face covered with a hat or hood, screaming for no apparent reason (since the light hurts their eyes), covering their eyes all the time, and avoiding things like televisions or movie theater screens. Another interesting condition I've noticed is that very often a sign of high manganese is very large pupils. Not always, but often enough to mention.

Over sensitivity to touch. This one is hard to bear for parents as it makes the children very reluctant to be touched. No hugging, no snuggling and frequently no breast feeding. They often want to take their clothes off, can only wear certain fabrics, or complain about tags or other irritants on their clothing. Often, the child can't keep any kind of covering on him or her in bed, causing very compromised and insufficient sleep as the poor things keep kicking off any covering, then get cold and pull it on, then kick it off again. It can be one reason why so many of the kids hate haircuts, as the little cut hairs are unbearable to them on their skin. It can also show up as a "texture" issue with foods, where they will only eat certain temperature or textures of foods.

Over sensitivity to sound. This one seems easy but it's more complex. The most common are covering their ears, complaining that everything is too loud, and not being able to focus except in a silent room. I began to notice an even stranger manifestation of this, especially in older children in a large number of cases. Many of these children have a perception that people including siblings, teachers, kids at school, even their own parents "hate them." Because their sensitivity to sound is so high, they tend to believe that everyone is yelling at them. Imagine if you went to work and everyone there yelled at you all day, every day. You'd start believing everybody hated you pretty quickly too. As such, this may result in kids acting "defiant" or "mean." In their minds, they're just defending themselves.

The over sensitivity to smell is not something I encounter as frequently, but if it is present, it's usually connected to food. They want to smell everything first, and often say that everything smells "rotten." If a food doesn't smell perfect, they will avoid eating it. I have seen this come up as an aversion to classrooms as well, since they can't stand the blend of odors present in ordinary classroom atmospheres.

Many of the children also have very active imaginations that can create anything from complicated imaginary worlds, to being unbelievably competent liars. Most common are extremely vivid dreams that encompass anything from a complex plot to horrific nightmares. I've had four-year-olds tell me nightmares they've had that gave me nightmares! I think the main reason for this one is because so many of these kids I've seen affected are authentically brilliant. You should see some of their IQs!

There is a pervasive school of thought recently (particularly among adults but I see it in kids too) that it is their autism itself that is "making them brilliant." I've received some very... shall we say... "colorful" letters and emails from people calling out my audacity for thinking that autism and ASD's are something that can and should be erased. Their fear is that if they are not affected by their autism, ADD, or whatever syndrome they have been diagnosed with, their "genius" will disappear with it. Well, rest easy folks because I can honestly say that I have never, not once in all my years, seen this to be the case. After the high manganese symptoms clear they remain bright and imaginative, but no longer out of control or frightened. What disappears is the overwhelming sensory input, anxiety, nightmares, and lack of focus. The brilliance (if it is indeed there) stays intact and can now become more clearly and easily utilized.

Although I'm focusing on the kids in this book, I do want to touch briefly on how Menefe Syndrome can affect adults. In adults the high sensory input causes many of the same responses that children have, but as adults we generally handle them differently. One of the major problems with adults is that they tend to ignore or deny that they have any issues going on until they become a huge problem. We ignore things like night terrors as "stress" for so long that they eventually become hallucinations. We ignore light and sound sensitivity and attribute our lack of attention to "being too busy."

One of the most aggravating symptoms I see in adults is a strange type of paranoia, or what I've come to call "The Worst Case Scenario." Kids will do this too sometimes, but it's much more prevalent in adults. These people will take what would normally be considered a small and insignificant occurrence, and keep adding more things that "could" have happened - but didn't - until they have a Jenga pile of anxiety built up. As an example, I had an adult man come to me because his blood pressure was getting high and he was developing little head tics. As it turned out his high manganese was causing paranoia, which was causing him to think he was losing his mind, which was causing him to be very anxious, which was causing his physical manifestations... you get my drift.

It remains truly amazing to me that the same high sensory in-put is able to manifest in so many forms. Autism in one, ADD in another, and anxiety and paranoia in yet another. The list I've seen of symptoms is mind blowing. And because this list encompasses a growing number of individuals, the Spectrum Balance® Protocol becomes increasingly relevant.

CHAPTER FIVE

Sources of Manganese

So if this Menefe Syndrome creates the symptom of high sensory input, why doesn't it all look the same? Why are there so many different ways in which it presents itself? I'll give you a metaphor I often use. Let's say that three people are sitting in a room as I explain Menefe Syndrome and the Spectrum Balance® Protocol and there are five television sets and five radios all blaring away on different stations. Person A is interested in baseball, and every time one of the stations mentions baseball, his focus shifts to listen to it in every case. Person B decides that she is going to focus on the TV set in front of her. She will block out all the rest of the input by becoming the world's expert on whatever is on that TV. And if you try to distract her from that, you better watch out! Person C can't take all the noise so she closes her eyes, covers her ears and sits in her own world blocking everything else out. So with all three of these people receiving exactly the same input, we have three completely different responses. Person A would most likely be diagnosed with ADD, Person B with Aspergers, and Person C with Autism. The exact same input causing multiple different symptoms, all because people simply have differing coping skills.

How much manganese you need a day seems to vary widely depending on who you ask. There are reports saying that 10 mg to 11 mg daily are the "tolerable," read "the most you can stand" level, with pretty extreme side effect warnings if you exceed that level. But since I'd hate to judge levels on what I can probably tolerate rather than what is good for me, I'm going to use the most common recommended limits for adults, which are in the 1.8 mg to 2.3 mg range for this discussion.

It is my belief that the prenatal environment plays a large role in the etiology of Menefe Syndrome, so let's look first at the dietary patterns of the mother. In today's world of rampant consumption of packaged, junk and fast food, we have to look at it as a component. So where is an expectant mom obtaining all this manganese? Some of the most likely suspects include:

1. High consumption of manganese-rich foods. See the "avoid" food list on the Protocol for many of these!

2. Regular consumption of high and/or cumulative doses of manganese from vitamins and other supplements. Check the labels of all the supplements you take and add up how many milligrams of manganese each has. Most people go way over the recommended 2 milligrams!

3. High consumption of phytate-rich foods, especially grains, that results in mineral imbalances and deficiencies, especially of iron.

4. Maternal anemia by any cause, which is proven to promote higher manganese absorption. Open iron receptor sites often equal high manganese, so if the mother's blood levels of manganese are high for any reason it can result in significantly greater levels in the developing fetus. And since manganese has been proven to actually concentrate through the umbilical cord this can cause a host of problems. Many "high quality" prenatal vitamins I've researched can contain as much as 300% of the daily recommended dosage for an adult. So if Mom is getting a 300% overdose, it is now concentrating in the umbilical cord and giving her baby, which may be only about the size of a sea monkey, a 450%

overdose *for an adult*. With the suggested dose for a baby being at 0.003% this is a bewilderingly massive overdose!

Another common source is the general poor digestive health of the mother. This can be from the presence of Candida and other yeast excess, improper absorption of nutrients in the gut, or even the chronic consumption of antacids. Or it could be that she's not eating whole real foods! Again, these factors are nearly all related back to diet.

One example that is not related to the mother's diet is when a newborn requires emergency medical intervention due to a premature birth or other health challenges. Although these intravenous nutrition treatments have saved many young lives, it is important to know that they are also very high in manganese. Again, with the recommended dose for a child from newborn to six years old being .003 mg, many of these IV fluids can contain as much as 25 mg per milliliter! The worst part is that this incurs much more damage at this stage since the child will absorb it at a higher rate because of his or her developing brain, and because he/she has not yet acquired proper liver function. Until a child has developed a mature biliary system and an intact blood-brain barrier they are at higher risk.

Once you have your baby home, there are new exposures:

1. Minimal or absence of breast feeding. Breast milk is the perfect food, and if the baby doesn't get it for whatever reason, he/she is starting at a deficit.

2. Not breast feeding also creates the need for using a formula of some kind, and nearly all of them are high in both phytates and manganese. Soy baby formulas, which were very much in use for a time, are the worst offenders.

3. Any dietary supplement that contains manganese. Any level may be too much!

These common factors may very well produce a nutritional pattern very early in life that overloads manganese and simultaneously provides excess levels of phytate and other anti-nutrients that prevent the availability of adequate levels of bio-available iron.

As your child gets older, even more sources become available as they begin to eat more solid and "baby foods" and their dietary patterns begin to change.

1. The regular consumption of high-manganese and high-phytate foods that are quite commonly marketed as "baby foods." One of the worst offenders is "teething biscuits." When I first began this research, the manganese levels, which were often in the overdose range for a single biscuit, were reported on the product label. Oddly, now I am unable to find a single brand that reports its manganese content on the label. Instead I see either "NA" or the symbol, ~. An FDA website explained that the mysterious symbol means that the manufacturer knows the amount of manganese -- but doesn't care to report it. Seriously, look it up! Why would they do that?

2. A huge contributing factor that I've seen is the transition to excessive consumption of cereal-based foods. Not only are these extremely high in phytate, they are often high in manganese as well. How often is baby's first food oatmeals and other cereals?

3. In the admirable quest to keep their kids healthy, parents often feel the need to give them children's vitamins. If you feel like this is something you really want to do, please be very cautious about these as many of them not only contain artificial colors and flavors (more anti-nutrients), but even the "good" (and expensive) ones can constitute a landslide of manganese.

4. And then of course there are the "healthy whole grains." It seems that "healthy whole grains" are in everything these days, doesn't it? The fact is that some of the very tip-top highest sources of manganese are in the "healthy whole grains" department. Choices like spelt, brown rice, soy and oats that have been touted for ages as "health foods" are among the worst offenders. Of course, these are all things that those of us who are already on a grain-free Paleo diet don't eat at all. And they are an absolute "no-no" on the Protocol!

There is also the case of diets that simply do not include sufficient levels of bio-available iron. This is especially indicated in the case of vegetarian or vegan lifestyles, as meat-source (heme) iron is several times more readily utilized in our bodies than is plant-source (non-heme) iron. Heme iron is also more resistant to chelation by dietary phytates than non-heme iron, so it has a tendency to stay more bio-available.

As much as I hesitate to step on the toes of what a parent wants to do, it is a plain fact. If you want your young child to be vegetarian or vegan, realize that they will be more susceptible to this iron/manganese imbalance, and therefore more likely to suffer the symptoms related to Menefe Syndrome.

We live in a fast food, junk food, packaged food world. When a child is eating a "bad" (junk food) or "SAD" (Standard American Diet) it is easier to think that their issues may be coming from what they are eating. But the fact is that even children on what are considered to be "good" diets are still being affected by massive rates of Autism Spectrum Disorders.

This is the beauty of the Spectrum Balance® Protocol. It's not just all about "good" or "organic" foods. **It's about the right foods to correct the iron and manganese imbalance**. As they say, it's all about the right tool for the right job.

6 - 10

Autism and related ASD's are definitely "equal opportunity offenders" as they strike children across the board. I have seen kids that were eating what has come to be known as the SAD (Standard American Diet) way; with lots of fast foods, packaged foods, and convenience foods be affected, and I have seen children with what is considered a "healthy" diet be hit just as hard. As it turns out, it was the actual foods themselves as much as the quality of the food that was the key.

When a child is eating mostly "junk" food it is easy to lay the blame on their poor dietary habits. But what do you say when a child who has had no vaccines, was breastfed, and has eaten nothing but a clean, whole, and organic diet is then diagnosed with an ASD?

As you know by now, The Spectrum Balance Protocol is a targeted Paleo diet. And it is that targeting of the iron and manganese imbalance that sets it apart from the standard Paleo diet. That sets it apart from any diet really.

The following case studies are some examples of kids who were affected not only by autism, but by a variety of ASD's, who were on what is nearly universally considered to be "healthy" diets. Organic, vegetarian and even (non-targeted) Paleo diets all fall into these categories. Including a little girl who was only eating *one food* that she shouldn't be that caused all her behavioral and developmental issues. One food…

CASE STUDY 6

Mom: *"He's just a ten-year-old now."*

Comments: Rx: none   DX: Autism @ 15 months

tx: 10 in June

On SBP

Note: His skin is vy yellowish .... leaky gut and of an absorption problem

Notes:

Has been dy luck batly since b; on SBP — "but it's time for for the next step"

Name: Dylan D. (Male)

Age: 10
DX: Autism
ND: Linda Kane
Other diets: GFCF

Sometimes it is easy to see where the high manganese has come from, such as the usual suspects of a soy baby formula or IV nutrition, and in other cases it's much more of a mystery. In this case of Dylan, he was breastfed for the first two years of his life, then put on very clean, organic and natural baby food. Yet at only fifteen months old, before he was even off breast milk, his parents could tell that something was wrong. He had received all of his vaccines so that was one possibility they were considering, but there was no easy answer on this one.

At fifteen months, Dylan still had no words; not even baby babble. He shunned any type of affection, even as a tiny baby, and actively disliked being touched. Often, distaste for affection is written off by the parents as part of that child's personality, and sometimes I think that's true. Some of us are just naturally more cuddly than others, but over the years I have come to see it as a symptom of the extreme sensory overload of touch. I don't see that one as frequently as light or sound sensitivities, but if it exists, it is usually quite severe. I've had lots of these kids say it physically hurts them when they are touched by a person, a blanket, a tag in the back of a shirt, the little hairs from getting a haircut, almost anything. He certainly fell into this category since something as simple as getting a haircut from his dad would send Dylan into screaming tantrums.

When you've seen as many of these cases as I have, some of the symptoms seem to start linking together. For example, in the kids I've worked with who "hate affection" I also find that nearly all of them have pretty extreme fears and paranoias. It makes me wonder if repulsion to being touched is more related to the pain it causes or to the claustrophobia of feeling closed in or smothered. Maybe a bit of both? I can say that in all the cases I've worked with, the kids do become at least more affectionate. Some of them turned into real cuddle monsters!

Within the autism world, there is a growing thought process that autistic kids are "just fine the way they are" and that we should "leave them alone and let them be who they are." I've even received some pretty scathing hate mail from adults with Aspergers for suggesting that autism is something that can (or should) be reversed. Let me say for the record here that I one-hundred percent disagree with that line of thinking! According to the affected kids I've spoken with, the majority of them were not fine; they were living in a nightmare world of overwhelming sensory input that caused their symptoms in the first place. Everything is too bright, too loud, too harsh, and they live with unrealistic fears of everyday things, terrible nightmares, and an inability to communicate. Doesn't sound "fine" to me! Dylan was one such child.

It was harder to find something Dylan was not afraid of than what he did fear. He was so terrified of the neighbor's small dog that he would sometimes scream and kick at it if he saw it. His combination of paranoia and claustrophobia would cause him a horrific amount of anxiety because he could never decide if he wanted someone with him or not. As his mom described it, he was in a constant tug-of-war of "Stay here. No go away. No stay here."

At age ten, he now had some words, but he couldn't organize them. As is the case with so many of the non-verbal or limited-verbal kids, the frustration of wanting to say something but being unable to was revealing itself through tantrums, yelling, and banging his head. Even as adults we can all relate to how frustrating it is when you can't organize your thoughts or find the right word. Imagine an entire lifetime of it.

On the advice of his ND, Dylan had already begun the Protocol prior to his appointment with me, and in only two weeks they had seen some very positive changes. He was picking up new words daily, and a few times had been able to string them together into a short sentence. His dad, preparing for the usual screaming rodeo of a haircut, was surprised when Dylan stayed calm and for the first time, actually seemed to enjoy it.

Seeing these changes so quickly inspired Dylan's mom to drive the multi-state trip to bring him in to see me. Her feeling was that if she was going to do this, she wanted to do it as perfectly as possible. I love that attitude as it not only shows commitment to her child, it means that I don't have to spend the entire time convincing her about the scientific background of the Protocol and can spend more time on the actual logistics of the diet.

As it turned out, there were some issues that needed sorting out in his diet. Although everything was whole, organic food, and were Protocol-approved foods, Dylan was eating far too much fruit and not nearly enough meats and good fats. As many kids his age are, he was a big sugar craver and ate way too many apples and dried mangoes. He did not like dairy (good!) but he also didn't like meat. His diet was primarily constituted of "fish, fruit, and veggies." While still in the office, his mom and I cruised through multiple internet Paleo cooking sites and were able to find him some recipe ideas that better balanced his proteins, fats and carbohydrates. It would take some creative work on her part but she was raring to go.

<u>One-month progress report : (phone)</u>

There was no doubt that the tweaks we had made to his diet were working, and working quickly. Dylan was suddenly showing a new calmness and maturity level that his parents had never seen before. In order to optimize the Protocol, Mom had needed to throw Dylan quite far out of many of his long-term dietary patterns, and he was adjusting like a champ. "He really understands some very mature things and he knows the diet is helping." I can't tell you how many times I have heard this statement over the years. Kids really do know what's good for them!

Dylan's communication skills were growing in some subtle and not so subtle ways. While his growing vocabulary and word organization were easily noticeable, Mom was finding it interesting that he was beginning to gesture more while he was speaking. Since Dylan had been taught sign language in his years of being non-verbal, I reminded her to make sure that he was using his words and not just signing them. This is often a problem with kids who sign, and their language skills can develop more slowly as a result. However, Mom assured me that he was not signing words, just trying to deliver more emotion and depth into his spoken words. Wow. She was right! That was a sure sign of growing maturity.

The subjects of his conversations had noticeably changed in character. Previously, his comments had consisted mostly of single words, usually to indicate things he wanted. He now was starting to comment on what other people were doing and had begun to ask questions. This was especially notable because autistic children will rarely if ever ask questions. In fact, it is often a device I use to detect improvement. If I can induce them to ask a question about me, they're making progress.

As it generally happens, the tantrums had stopped as soon as he was able to communicate more fully. He had one entire day when he was apparently a real Tasmanian devil, then it just stopped. Having a real whopper of a bad day like that before settling down is actually quite common. Although some kids' bad behavior will taper off, it is much more usual with the Protocol to see them have an extremely bad day or two and then just stop. Maybe they're just better than we "smart" adults at tossing out bad habits!

The irrational and terrifying fears that Dylan had been suffering from his entire life were quickly fading away. When I asked about them, his mom explained, "It's not fear. More like he's emotional sometimes." With the absence of the gnawing paranoia and claustrophobia, Dylan was able to begin finding happiness and peace in being alone. He was settling down and doing his homework with no battles when he was asked to, he was playing independently for the first time in his life, and he was becoming quite the Lego architect. After not seeing him for awhile one night, his mother went to check on him in his room where he was busy changing all the tires on his toy trucks. "It was time," he informed her seriously.

One area that was proving harder for him was that he was on the affection roller coaster. He just couldn't figure out what he wanted to do. He'd run out and hug his mom or dad then run back in his room. That was okay, he'd figure it out in time. As Mom observed, "Poor guy. All of his years of being non-emotional are happening all at once."

As I always did at the end of a phone consultation, I asked his mother what was new, or what was her favorite thing that happened in this last month. This phrase may not seem like much if you don't have an autistic child, but if you do it will speak volumes: "He has his own will now. He used to just do what I said."

Two-month progress report: (phone)

This month had brought even more changes, and Mom was very happy and excited at all his new gains. "Our only issue is communication. Other than that, he's just a little boy now."

The hyperactivity that had once been uncontrollable was now just "boundless boy energy." Dylan was happy and healthy and gaining height and muscle tone. The growing maturity that was hinted at before was now evident in his new grown-up behaviors. Instead of being a "picky little kid," he was now eating a wider variety of foods, and asking to try foods they'd never had before. He was becoming open to new experiences and was asking to visit new places, like the park or especially to a baseball game. He was willing to take the few supplements he was on, and was sticking to the diet on his own volition -- a behavior I'd like to see more of in my adult clients. He began showing his new independence by starting to cut up his own food at mealtimes, and by initiating chores such as putting away groceries or setting the table without being asked. In short, Dylan was finding his own way.

Although communication was still the parents' sticking point, Dylan was making successful strides with his speech. In the last month his pronunciation had become much sharper, and they noticed that even the sound of his voice had become more tonal and mature. When frustrated, he would fall back on sign language from time to time, but the whole family had trained themselves to gently ask him use his words. As a result, he was speaking with enhanced clarity and with more full sentences.

Dylan's irrational fears of "nearly everything" had seen the most noticeable change. He could still be a "bit emotional" at times, but his parents had identified the trigger as him being very tired. How many of us can relate to that? In this short period of time Dylan had progressed from being "frightened of everything" to "wary of some things." This was very solid progress and I felt certain that it would continue to improve.

He still wasn't quite sure which side of the affection fence he wanted to be on yet. While he was much more social in general, and was asking questions about other people, he was still a bit on the shy side. His parents were very willing to let him figure this out for himself, and I was happy to hear it. His Mom said, "He's so funny now and he's such a tease." Good enough for now.

Three-month progress report: (phone)

This month Dylan made his decision about the whole "being affec-tionate" thing. He was in. His mom said that all of a sudden his desire for affection just burst out. "It's very much and very cute. He's quite huggy and sweet and he loves to high-five people." It started out with the immediate family first, with him wanting to hug them and help them do things. I guess he liked how it made him feel, because pretty soon the babysitter was getting her share, with Dylan hugging her and telling her that he "loves her." Worlds away from his former fearful isolationist behavior, he was now seeking out a neighbor who jogs by his house so they could have their daily high five. He was creating new games himself, and asking others to play them with him. Life was becoming happier for him and his family.

"It's like having a normal life" his Mom explained. "Yesterday, he just held me for a long time. He hasn't done that since he was a baby."

His communication at this point was progressing strongly, with constant steady improvement. While still needing some more speech therapy, both the family and their ND felt that he was doing "spectacularly well." There was no doubt that while he was still having trouble with certain words, he fully understood everything that was being said to him, and he was doing his part and obviously trying his best.

When I asked what the best or newest improvements were this month, they had a lot to choose from. "Dylan has had lots of growth in education, maturity and relationships. He wants to try new foods and asks if he can try them. His schoolwork is great, and he's singing the theme songs to shows he watches. I never thought we'd get here."

Dylan was also growing ever more independent and had shocked his parents by asking if he could have his own room. "Only a few months ago he was terrified of the dark. He has his own bedroom now and is very excited about it. He would have been so scared before and now he loves it."

Dylan was rapidly catching up and becoming a "regular" ten-year-old, and both he and his family were happy.

Four-month progress report: (phone)

We were now at the four-month mark, and all was going extremely well. His normally very chatty mom, who always took notes so she could remember what she wanted to tell me (bless her), didn't have as much to say today. "He's very ten and he likes to goof around,"

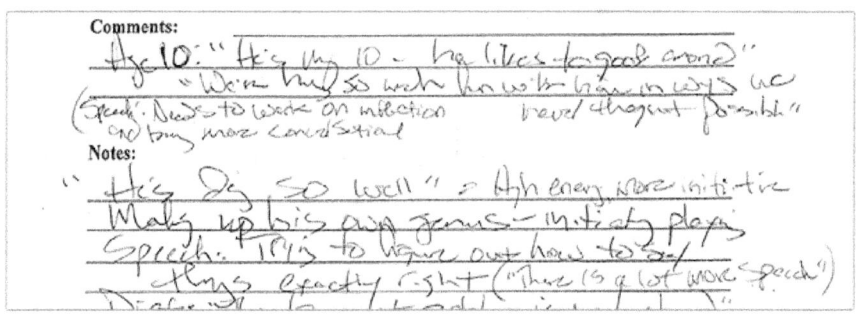

she laughed. "We're having fun with him now in ways that we would have never thought possible."

The only need for improvement left was for Dylan to catch up on his speech. "He has a lot more speech. He's just trying to figure out how to say things perfectly now." The three groups that constituted his team on this; his parents, his ND, and myself, all agreed that it would simply take time. He had a lot of non-verbal years to catch up to.

Dylan was loving his new man cave, although his parents were still a bit shocked that he not only wanted it but was so happy in a room of his own. He was meticulously (but not obsessively) keeping it neat and tidy and was obviously proud of having his own space. The paralyzing fears that he had dealt with most of his life had already faded into memory, and a new independence was growing in their place.

His parents began a very significant change by giving him options regarding discipline. This way he would clearly understand that if he's going to do something outside the family rules, he's going to have to pay the piper. If he did something he knew he shouldn't have (like any kid), they would ask him, "Do you want to go to your room or do you want to stand in the corner?" He was then able to choose his particular punishment, and would then calmly submit to it. This was teaching him clearly that there are consequences to our actions, and personally I wish more people would do this with their kids. But more importantly, this kind of thought process and choice making are considered impossible for an autistic person. Dylan was no longer just his diagnosis, and his family knew it. They were treating him for what he was, a ten-year-old boy, and he was rising to every challenge.

After a lull in the conversation, I asked his mom my usual question. What did she feel was left that we needed to work on? She had to give it some serious thought, then answered, "I guess he needs to catch up on his speech some, but he's doing great. He's… just a ten-year-old boy now".

Follow-up:

In September, 2011, I discharged Dylan on a regular Paleo diet, with an eye to the "avoid list" of high manganese foods from the Protocol. It's funny how people will refer to autistic kids as "special" when what most of the kids themselves really want is just to be like everyone else. Dylan got his wish.

CASE STUDY 7

Mom: *"She's always eaten organic, whole grains, whole foods, gluten free and vegetarian."*

Name: Bailey M. (Female)

Age: 3
DX: None officially
Other diets: "Healthy whole grains," tofu, pasta, all organic, vegetarian
Note: No vaccines

Although Bailey was not officially diagnosed with anything, this short case study very clearly makes so many of my points for me, I decided to include it. **If your child, whether they are three or thirty, has some bizarre unexplainable behaviors, I would encourage you to continue reading.**

Point 1: Being in denial that something is wrong is not going to help your child.

At only three years old, Bailey had such extreme anger issues that she was very nearly uncontrollable. What had begun as a major inconvenience had escalated into an actual physical violence issue. Her fits and tantrums were now becoming so rampant that they constituted a danger to her siblings as she was starting to hit, scratch, and bite during her tirades. Despite this, her mom was in complete denial about her child's behavior, insisting that Bailey was "just going through a phase." Fortunately the toddler's grandma, a long time client of mine and a clinical psychologist, was there at the appointment to set the record straight. While she was trying to explain what Bailey's "fits" looked like, the girl's mother kept saying, "Oh, Mom, don't exaggerate. They're not that bad."

Just as I was wondering how I was going to be able to get to the truth of the matter, Bailey launched into a screaming, howling fit! Not exaggerating, it looked like something out of a scary movie, and there was no visible trigger. For no reason anyone could discern she suddenly went stiff as a board as if she were having a seizure, then started screaming bloody murder. Her now crying mother and determined grandma were having quite the struggle just trying to hold her still. Thrashing wildly now, Bailey got loose and grabbed a handful of the pencils, pens and scissors that were in a pencil holder on my desk. Before anyone could react, she then flung them across the desk directly at my face. I ducked reflexively, but most of the pens and pencils hit me, and the scissors actually cut my cheek just under my left eye. In my many years of working with "special needs" kids, I've been hit, kicked and bitten by a few, but this is the only one who almost did real harm.

While I went to stop the bleeding on my cheek, the ladies worked on calming her down. By the time I went back in, Bailey was sitting on the floor humming to herself as if there was no one else in the room, and nothing had happened. Her mom was still crying, but I think her grandma was relieved to know that I now knew the truth.

The weirdest part of all of this was that these fits and other behavioral problems were not even what she was brought in about! That just goes to show you how powerful denial can be.

Point 2: A "healthy diet" may not be the right diet.

Of all the most common schools of thought about what causes autism, Bailey had none of them. No one in her family tree had any kind of ADD or autism issues that they knew about, she was breastfed for sixteen months, and she had received no vaccines. Boom, boom, and boom. What else you got?

Her mom's first concern, amazingly, since I had just witnessed (and was still bleeding from) one of her "fits," was for her digestive problems. "Bailey has never had a single firm poop in her life," I was told. She had literally, since birth, had nothing but diarrhea. In addition, at just under a year old while still being only breastfed strangely enough, she began developing horrible allergies. Her eyes and nose would swell up and run, and she would get rashes on her hands and arms. Now, two years later, she was still experiencing them.

When I asked about her diet, her mom waved it off. "It can't be that. She's always eaten organic, whole grains, whole foods, and vegetarian. And I always have too."

And there it was. "Healthy" whole grains, tofu, soy -- and no meats. Although I shy away from criticizing whatever lifestyle people choose to adopt, in this case I had to step in. The fact is that vegetarians are massively more prone to Menefe Syndrome than are omnivores (those who eat both plant-based foods and meat). Typically, in order to get full without eating meats and healthy fats, vegetarians usually want to load up on breads, potatoes, pastas, rice, and "meat substitutes" that are generally made from soy. With all the grains she was eating chelating the iron and leaving those receptor sites available, coupled with the massive amount of manganese that is in soy, it was no wonder that Bailey was affected.

As you can imagine, explaining the idea that Bailey would need to start eating meat, good fats, and (gulp) absolutely no grains was not going over well with her mom. "Meat? That's disgusting!" she wailed. "I haven't touched meat since I was sixteen." She also baked her own whole grain wheat bread daily, and the family generally ate more than a loaf a day. That explained a lot because truthfully, I was questioning what Mom's own manganese levels might look like. Starting off with the complete denial that Bailey's violent tantrums were "just a phase," during the course of the appointment she cried off and on, and displayed a constant hand wringing anxiety.

And so is revealed yet another of the major roadblocks to the Protocol being more universally practiced. Since the imbalance is caused by diet, and families most commonly all eat the same meals, it is not unusual for one or both of the parents to be affected as well, with or without a diagnosis. It is far, far, far from unusual for me to see an autistic child who has a bipolar, ADD or schizophrenic parent or parents. As this Protocol constitutes a very significant change in lifestyle for most people, I have had any number of moms tell me that it was "more than they could handle," and never even attempted it. There are even some dads (more than you can imagine) who "forbid" the family from being on the Protocol because they so adamantly do not wish to change their diets. And if they aren't gonna do it, well then darn it, no one will.

There is no doubt in my mind that this would have been one of those cases where there was never even an attempt made. At the thought of eating meat and not eating oatmeal every morning, Mom was in tears again. Fortunately for Bailey, it was grandma to the rescue! Since she was a long time client of mine and was therefore already eating according to my guidelines, she offered to cook and feed Bailey all her meals. Mom heaved a dramatic sigh and agreed that under those circumstances they could give it a try.

Point 3: The Spectrum Balance Protocol IS a gut-healing diet!

One of the questions that Bailey's mom had was whether she should start immediately onto the Protocol, or if she needed a "gut healing diet" first. I've had this question many times, and the answer is no. Enough said…

One-month progress report:

Even though my cheek had healed, I was wary enough when I saw her name on my appointment list a month later that I took anything that could be used as a projectile off my desk. As it turned out there was no need.

Bailey was smiling, happy and sweet today. She politely asked if she could borrow my colored pens (the same ones she had thrown at me last time), and drew me a little picture. Mom said she was "doing great" and was enthusiastic about the changes. "This is an unbelievable change! She's turned into such a cuddly and sweet child. Everyone notices."

To the relief of her entire family, she had not had a single tantrum or fit for nearly three weeks. In the place of her anger, Bailey was showing an innate sweetness that no one had anticipated. "She's very approachable, cuddly, and happy."

The change in diet had also brought around a nearly immediate change in her digestive problems as well. "She's having firm poops for the first time in her life," Mom reported proudly. Although not a particular fan of extended poop conversations, I was happy to hear that her poor tortured tummy had settled down, and that the diarrhea, the allergies, and the rashes had all disappeared.

When I asked her mom how she herself was doing on the Protocol, she immediately snapped, "Oh I'm not on it. The kids are, but I could never give up my whole grain breads and oatmeal." Despite realizing that since she had started eating that way when she was sixteen so her grain-eating habit was, well, ingrained, still I was shocked! I asked her how she could have just witnessed what the Protocol could do in one short month with the once-terrorizing Bailey yet remain so opposed to trying it for herself? She got very rattled and kept repeating, "I just can't. I just can't do it. I can't give up bread" like a mantra. Not surprisingly she had worked herself into tears again at this point. Bailey tried to comfort her, but her grandma stared silently down at her crossed hands in her lap. Apparently I wasn't the only one who wished Mom would try the Protocol for herself.

Going from her Linda Blair-style tantrum the previous month, Bailey was now easily the calmest person in the room. Her mom was in high anxiety, and you could feel the waves of frustration coming off of Grandma (a psychologist, remember), and I was in utter shock. How could someone watch her child go from an uncontrollable screaming mess to an angel in thirty days and not immediately want to try that for themselves? Now, this was back in 2006 when things still shocked me. Not so much these days. In the following years I would see this exact attitude scores of times. Now instead of shock it just makes me feel sad.

Trying hard to comfort her crying mom, Bailey broke the rather tense silence by taking her hand and saying, "C'mon, Mommy. You need to go home." As they headed down the stairs, Grandma and I sat in silence. There was a lot not being said in that room. Finally she looked up from her clasped hands and sighed. "I'll keep Bailey on the Protocol. I have the kids most of the time anyway."

As she started to go, I couldn't help chiming in, even though family politics are certainly none of my business. "You know, if she would just…" I didn't get any further. I guess it was an old conversation and Grandma was sick of it. She held a hand up to me, and I stuttered to a stop. Another lesson learned: You can't fix everyone.

Follow-up:

At no surprise to me, I did not hear from them for eight months. When her mom called in asking an unrelated health question, I asked how Bailey was faring. Her response seemed a bit … something. Evasive? Dismissive? Very quickly she responded, "Oh, she's just an amazing cuddle bug" and got off the phone. Huh.

Several years later I was having an appointment with Bailey's big sister, who had a sore throat and would not willingly see any other doctor than me. She's a believer! The whole time Bailey was lying on the floor of my office coloring in a book and humming. When I'd look down at her she would shoot me a big smile, and once a blown kiss. I don't know why it is the case, but some of the most wild and extreme kids that I have seen are also often the cutest ones. As I looked down at her blond curls and big blue eyes, it was hard to equate this angelic visage with the kid who had thrown my own scissors in my face.

As her mom handed her some crayons I observed, "It's amazing the transformation in Bailey, isn't it"? Not meeting my eyes, she said, "I don't know what you mean."

What? What do you mean, what do I mean? Uh, the screaming fits, the anger, the digestive problems? The throwing sharp objects at me? With all this going through my mind, I settled for saying "Uh. Her behavioral issues?"

Mom sat there and completely disavowed that anything had ever been wrong with Bailey. Despite the older daughter siding with me ("Mommy, it was too!"), she insisted, "That wasn't Bailey. She was never like that. You're thinking of the wrong child."

No, I wasn't. When a three-year-old nearly puts your eye out, you remember her! Given that Mom denied anything was wrong in the first place I guess I shouldn't have been so surprised. But it brings me to:

Point 4: Denial that anything was ever wrong isn't helping either.

If you don't learn from your mistakes you are destined to repeat them. And it certainly doesn't help get the word out about the Protocol that may dramatically help the many thousands of people of all ages to enjoy a glowing state of robust wellness. Had this mother put Bailey back on her original grain-intensive diet, the chances are high that all of her symptoms would have reappeared over time.

In this case, Bailey lucked out. Her family moved back east shortly after my last conversation with her mom, and her grandma (dear, amazing Grandma) moved with them. She is Paleo and has kept the kids on the straight and narrow. After all these years, she still has been unable to get her own daughter on the Protocol, or even on Paleo. It breaks her heart, so we don't talk about it much. As I said, you can't save everyone, but I'm sure it hurts more when it's your own daughter. Adults or not, they're still your kids.

CASE STUDY 8

Mom: *"Her tests from school were off the charts!"*

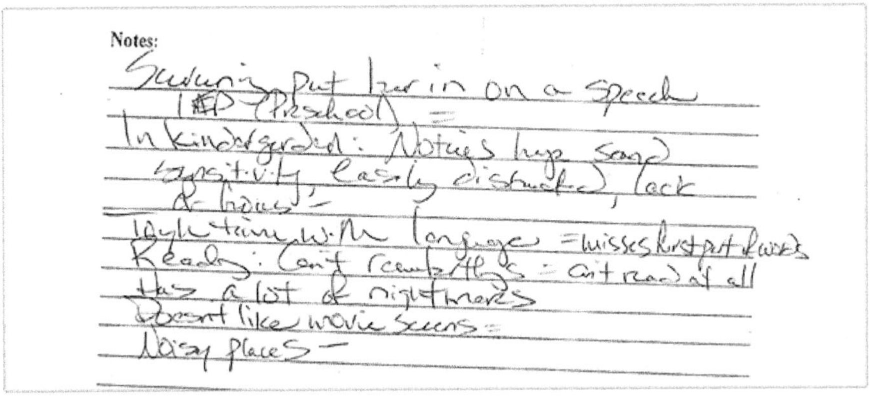
Notes:
Screening put her in on a speech
IEP (Preschool)
In kindergarten: Notices huge sound sensitivity, easily distracted, lack of focus
Tough time with language = misses first part of words
Reading: Can't remember things = can't read at all
Has a lot of nightmares
Doesn't like movie scenes
Noisy places

Name: Cate D. (Female)

Age: 6
DX: None officially. School tests put her in "special needs" speech therapy
Other diets: Paleo/Primal

As tempting as it is to show just the autism cases, I wanted to show a much larger range of symptoms that this Menefe Syndrome imbalance can cause. Though not officially DX'd Cate's symptoms are so common and not something that is generally linked to a particular syndrome or problem. How many kids who are having trouble with reading, comprehension, and speech are linked to high manganese levels? That's why I suggest people just try the diet for a few months and see what happens even if your child is not diagnosed with anything or is showing "autism symptoms."

It is important to note that Cate was already on a Paleo/Primal diet (no grains, limited dairy). This targeted approach of the Spectrum Balance Protocol for a few months was what she needed in order to correct the mineral balance and break through.

Hard as I try to not have favorites, sometimes you just can't help it. Cate is just such a funny and truly special kid. Most kids just want to be "normal," whatever that looks like, but Cate was aiming for something much more lofty than that. She wanted to excel, and I admired her ambition. So much grit in such a little girl.

Cate's mom was a long-time client of mine, which was why the family was already Paleo. Cate was so smart and funny that they didn't even notice anything was wrong until she started school. They did know that she had a very low tolerance for any kind of noise, and that she hated movie screens, but as it so often is, these abnormal characteristics were just dismissed as sensitive hearing and vision.

Looking for clues, I asked Cate about the number-one most common symptom -- nightmares. Turns out that she was having very frequent and very vivid nightmares. Since she hadn't told her parents about them, they had not factored them in as part of a bigger problem. When her mom asked why she had never told them about the nightmares, Cate just said "They're not things I want to talk about."

Cate had an unusual way of speaking that I had never encountered. She obviously knew what she wanted to say, and you could mostly tell what she was saying, but she seemed to miss the first part of many words. The second and third syllables came out, but not the first one. In most cases I would suggest that she get her hearing checked, but in her case her hearing was obviously extremely sensitive and definitely not lacking. It was clear that she was embarrassed by this and didn't do much talking at our first session unless I asked her a question. I could tell from the words she was trying to say that there was nothing wrong with her vocabulary, it was all in the delivery.

As soon as Cate started kindergarten it was quickly noticed that she was easily distracted and was having a rough time focusing her attention, even though it seemed like she was trying. Although she desperately wanted to read, she just couldn't manage it. All her hard work was resulting in lots of frustrated tears but no new reading skills. For some reason she wasn't able to absorb what was being taught, and then she couldn't remember anything afterward. Poor kid, she really was trying so hard and it wasn't paying off.

Mom told me privately before their appointment that Cate had suffered a fairly severe closed head brain trauma at age two. She was afraid that these learning issues might be a consequence, but hesitated saying anything to Cate. I suggested she hold off telling her until we could see if the Protocol was going to work first. She was relieved to not have that conversation, and agreed.

Since her whole family was already Paleo, the Protocol was an easy matter of a few changes here and there. Her Mom was fascinated by the idea that a simple mineral imbalance could cause such weird symptoms, but was eager to get started. "I'm putting all of us on this. I think we could all use some better focus".

As I always do with school-age children, I spoke to Cate about the absolute necessity for her to be responsible about staying on the Protocol herself. With all the cupcake days and plethora of junky snack food at school, not to mention the school lunches themselves, there was plenty of temptation to fall off the wagon. While I was explaining this to her, she listened with an adult-like seriousness. This was my first clue that there was quite a brain ticking away in there. She didn't say much, but she was definitely listening. When I asked if she felt that was something she could do, she nodded very slowly and seriously, and said, "I'll take care of it."

<u>One-month progress report:</u>

Within the first ten days of the Protocol they were already noticing a definite change in the sensory input issues. Since her classroom sounded like a classroom now instead of a chainsaw factory, Cate was finding it much easier to settle down and focus. Although she was still having a hard time reading, they were finding that she could at least understand the concept of what she was working on and she was making progress. Her speech was going down the same path and she now understood that she was dropping the first syllable of words and was working on that herself.

Cate's mom was happy that she was sleeping so much better, and that the awful, vivid nightmares were no longer waking her. "I'm really glad about that too," added Cate. Mom also felt that the more restful sleep was having a large impact on her ability to focus as well. Personally, I think that one goes for everyone.

With all the wonderful progress Cate was making, her mom was very surprised to get a call from the school; she was told that Cate's teachers were concerned because she was not eating or drinking "anything." Their definition of "anything" turned out to be a bit skewed as Cate ate all her home-packed food, she just didn't eat the school food. It was Cate's refusal to indulge in the birthday cupcakes and lemonade that another child in the class had brought that day that had caused the concern.

At this point Cate --not her mom, Cate -- informed them that she was currently on a "special diet" and would not be eating anything that was not allowed on it. "I promised that I would not cheat on my diet, so I'm not going to." Well then. I guess she told them!

Although I'm not sure on what authority it did this, the school demanded to see this "so-called diet" Cate was on. Her mom brought a copy of it when she picked her daughter up from school the next day, and unfortunately, the school authorities thought it was ridiculous. No grains? No milk? Not even eating cupcakes? Surely her child would be become horribly stigmatized! They apparently debated this for quite awhile. Mom even offered to call me while she was there to answer any questions they may have had, but they were not interested. They knew better.

In the end, the school realized that it was just going to have to deal with it, because the final arbiter of this deal was not going to be the school, or even her parents. It was going to be Cate and that was that. The little girl stood her ground and I admire that. As her mom said to the school authorities, "Cate really stays after her diet. Good luck trying to get her to change her mind." Like I said, the girl's got grit.

Her school didn't like it, but was just going to have to deal with it. Tells you what a crazy topsy-turvy world we live in when a school is so concerned that a child doesn't want to eat sugar, and soda and other garbage that it demands a parent conference! The whole time through this process while Cate was so rapidly improving, the school kept fighting with her mom. Unfortunately for the school, it had come up against a wall. A six-year-old wall, named Cate.

At this point I suggested that Cate move from the strict Phase 1 part of the Protocol, and start incorporating more of the Phase 2 vegetables and fruit. As all three of us looked over a list of these new Phase 2 foods together, Cate gave her input as to which of them she would like to have first. She was very interested in trying some new things that she had never eaten before, and asked me what my favorites were and what they tasted like. We created several new recipes that were "Cate approved."

<u>Two-month progress report:</u>

This appointment was one of the most surreal experiences I have ever had in my life. This was a whole new kid! After very solemnly shaking my hand, Cate informed her mother that she wanted to start the appointment by herself and asked her to "Please wait here downstairs for a little while." Mom was startled, but agreed. Obviously, we two had something to discuss. I was intrigued.

Many parents have told me that one of the biggest reasons that their kids like me is because I take them seriously. I don't baby talk them in any way, shape, or form, and I make them personally responsible. I treat them more like small adults, and I give them my respect.

Having said this, I have to tell you that this was about the hardest I ever had to try to keep a straight face. Just the ladylike way that Cate settled into her chair told me that she had something of note on her mind, and that I better have my matching game face on. I folded my hands on my desk, put on a serious but interested expression on my face, and waited.

As she started to talk to me, I was immediately astounded at her speech! The quality of it had completely changed. Between that and her very advanced and adult-sounding vocabulary, it made me feel as if tea and crumpets should be involved somewhere in this process. Apparently, speaking correctly wasn't enough for her; she was now speaking elegantly and eloquently.

You have to understand that this girl, or little lady I should say, is so cute she looks like she just fell off a Victorian Valentine's Day card. It was an unbelievable trial to keep a poker face as I listened to this extremely adult language coming from the mouth of a six-year-old cherub, but I was not about to give her anything less than the respect she worked so hard for and heartily deserved.

Cate wanted to tell me about the recent trip her family had made to Disneyland. Apparently her mom had told her that I am originally from the Anaheim area and she wanted to compare notes on how it had changed since I was her age. It was hard to believe that her memory had ever been a problem, as she rattled off the names of all the rides, her favorite parts of the park, and where and what they had eaten. I asked her if she felt that it was harder to stay on the Protocol while they were on vacation, but she just shrugged dismissively and said, "I did really well. I know everything I can eat and that's what I eat." From the mouths of babes. She made it sound so simple.

"The reason I asked to speak with you alone," she explained, drawing something out of her purse, "is because I bought you a present at Disneyland with my own money. Since you're from there I thought you might like it."

Walking over to my desk, she laid a small, pink Tinkerbell stamp in front of me. Before I could respond she continued, "I felt Tinkerbell was appropriate for you since I think people should believe in you more." From a six-year-old! Okay kid, you're killing me. Straight face, straight face…

Pulling it together, I responded in the English Country House manner that she seemed to be striving for herself. "I would have appreciated anything from Disneyland, but I have always had a particular fondness for Tinkerbell. Thank you, Cate. I will cherish this." She gave me a smile and a graceful nod, then went down to fetch her mother for the rest of the appointment.

After our surreal trip to Woodworthy Manor, the rest of the appointment when Mom joined us was more brass tacks. Cate's new tests from school were "off the charts" including in spelling and comprehension. She was reading like crazy, including some books about British children who solve crimes around their country homes. Ah. That solved the mystery of the elegant wording she was using. Reading was her new joy and she was reveling in her newfound skills so much that she was writing her own book that used both words and pictures for extra credit in school. Her mother was beaming with pride, but Cate was taking it in stride. "Oh, I'm really good at everything now. Doing so good in school makes me really happy." Makes me happy too.

As I always do, I suggested that we make another one-month appointment to make sure all the changes were holding. They had been slowly expanding the foods they were currently eating, and we wanted to ensure that there was no regression.

As we stood to go, I again thanked Cate for her lovely gift. Her mom was surprised at that since she had not even known that she had brought me something. When I showed her what it was, you could see the immense pride welling up in her eyes. She finally managed, "Dr. Shauna's right, Cate. That is lovely." I got another formal handshake from Cate and she headed down the stairs. Her mom and I just looked at each other. What was there to say? We finally just allowed ourselves a quiet laugh and followed Her Ladyship down the stairs.

Three-month progress report:

A month later, all systems were still firmly a go. Cate's reading and comprehension skills continued to soar, and some new tests showed "over the top" math skills, as well as an "exceedingly high" score for computer skills. She was a learning machine now and there was no stopping her.

Apparently, she was still reading the British country house books. When I asked her if she was happy with her new lack of dietary restrictions as they transitioned back to Paleo, she said she felt there was a lot of new things that she was enjoying. "Cantaloupe is really good. Do you care for it?"

Follow-up:

I discharged Cate on a standard Paleo diet in June of 2011. Since her mom is a regular client of mine, I also get to see Cate from time to time. She's ten now, and she is exceptional. All her school scores remain exceedingly high and apparently, she's making computers do things people didn't know computers could do. She ditched the British mannerisms and ladylike speech somewhere along the way, and is more into rolling her eyes at me these days. To tell you the truth, I kind of miss it. I remember those conversations like they were yesterday; I'll never forget them! What a hoot.

By the way, I wasn't kidding or just being polite about cherishing my Tinkerbell stamp. She gave it to me more than three years ago, and I'm looking at it right now. Wherever I'm working, Tink goes with me. It's wonderful when someone believes in you. It's even more special when it's such a precious child.

CASE STUDY 9

Mom: *"We've accomplished all our goals. We're all good!"*

Notes:
Has been on SBP 4/30/10 = on Prss~3
now
[redacted] helps that it has recovided)
all their goals / "we're all good)"
look: Long term " for the rest of his
(like kind) of stuff."

Name: Dean K. (Male)

Age: 12
DX: Autism
Other diets: Kosher
ND: Michael Kane

Generally with these kids, there is a "before" and an "after" attached to their situation. In the case of Dean, all I saw was the "after." This was yet another family who decided to take matters into their own hands by starting the Protocol without initial consultation with me, so they had been on it for five months prior to coming into my office.

When the family (both parents this time; I rarely see fathers) came in and sat down, I was a bit mystified as to why they were there. It's rather unusual in a doctor's office to see everyone looking so happy, yet there they all were, beaming away at me. They had filled out my paperwork pertaining to kids on the autism spectrum, but in my initial observation of Dean sitting there, he was obviously not autistic. He was friendly, bright, chatty, and obviously extremely intelligent right from the get go; he greeted me with the charm and the courtly manners of the Southern gentleman that he is. I looked at the paperwork where I ask parents to rank their children's symptoms on a scale of zero to ten and all I saw was series of zeros. When I asked why they were here, Dean immediately piped up. With a sunny smile he said, "Oh, I used to be autistic."

And sure enough, he had been. At age six, when the family had adopted him from the Ukraine, he had already been diagnosed. I've seen quite a few times where a "special needs" child has been adopted, and the overwhelming love and generosity it takes to willingly take on a child like this never ceases to amaze me. No family that is expecting a baby actually hopes that they will have an autistic child, although they accept the idea as a possibility. These people willingly and consciously take these children into their lives and into their hearts knowing for a fact that there will be additional problems, and yet they do it anyway. Amazing.

At the time that they had decided to start the Protocol, appointments with me were being booked quite far in advance; often several months in advance especially for a Saturday. The first available one that worked with their travel schedule and mine was five months away, although being "autism parents" they were used to waiting. My front desk, when booking the appointment, suggested that they go ahead and start the Protocol before coming in, but alas, Dean's whole family was already enthusiastically on Phase 1 thanks to their ND, Michael Kane.

There was no doubt that his original diagnosis had been correct. Up until the last five months of his life, Dean had been hyperactive and irrational, with many developmental delays, and the usual suspects of sensory issues and nightmares. He often spent whole days "in his own world" and could not be brought out. In other words, he was a "textbook" case of autism. Looking at him now it was almost impossible to believe, but it was Dean himself who made the most compelling case.

Dean taught me a lot about what it is like to actually be autistic. It was difficult to listen professionally and unemotionally as he described his horrifying nightmares, the lack of connection to anything or anyone, and the constant onslaught of sensory input. Unlike most children, he not only remembered the irrational and frightening things he'd done, he even remembered why he did them and was eloquent in his explanations. It was fascinating.

Although many kids on the Spectrum have an over-sensitivity to pain, Dean's was nearly non-existent. He was always covered with bumps and bruises and would throw himself into dangerous situations where he could have been hurt without a thought. It was difficult to watch his dad's face when Dean described in detail an incident where his father had caught him trying to slice through his own thumb lengthwise with a large kitchen knife. I asked if he was purposely trying to hurt himself, to which he responded, "No. I knew it wouldn't hurt. I just wanted to see what a bone looked like."

Dean was very grateful that the nightmares had stopped only three weeks into the Protocol, as he had experienced them as long as he could remember. His mom knew he was getting better when a few weeks after starting the Protocol she playfully poked him on the arm with a pencil while they were doing homework and he reacted with "Ow! Stop it!" That may not seem like much to most people, but when you are constantly watching your son to make sure he doesn't cut himself with butcher knives or otherwise harm himself it speaks volumes!

Because of the advice and testimonials of their ND, the family had leaped enthusiastically into the Protocol; ridding the house of anything that didn't belong the same day they downloaded their copy,

To Noises / Sound? (0) 1 2 3 4 5 6 7 8 9 10
Includes jumping or reacting to abrupt noises, dislike of television, radios, etc., has an aversion
to movie theaters, complains that classrooms are "too noisy", often puts their hands over their
ears, complains that everyone is "yelling at them" Stopped 4 mos into Spectrum Protocol.

To Touch? (0) 1 2 3 4 5 6 7 8 9 10
Doesn't like the feel of tags in the back of clothing , the feel of certain clothes, doesn't like
sheets or blankets on them, is often too hot or too cold, dislikes haircuts, complains of skin
sensitivities or "creepy crawly" feeling, dislikes being touched or hugged Spectrum Protocol.
Stopped 2 weeks ago. 4 ½ months into
Claustrophobia? 0 1 2 3 4 5 6 7 8 9 10

and began strictly on Phase 1. "I just folded over the page to the
'Best' foods and made that my shopping list!" Mom recounted. They
had no trouble getting Dean to eat whatever they wanted him to simply because he had no opinion or even very much awareness of what
he was eating in the beginning. Even with the added restriction of
the family being kosher, they did not let that prevent or impede them
from trying a way of eating that held hope for their son. Now that
Dean had more input on how they were eating, he remained happy
with the Protocol. "There's meat and fat on it, so I'm good!" Spoken
like a true guy.

In the course of them waiting for their appointment, it had come to
their attention that although the Spectrum Balance Protocol was a
targeted approach, it was also a Paleo diet. Wanting to do his own
research, Dean had read "The Paleo Solution" by Robb Wolf, and
like so many other young men, he felt that "it resonated" with him.
We discussed the need for him to be careful with the high-manganese foods, which he said made him feel funny anyway, but I felt he
was ready to do the more mainstream (although kosher) Paleo diet.
Being that he felt strong, happy and was growing like a weed, he was
cool with that idea.

This appointment, which took place at the end of 2011, will always
live in my memory for several reasons. For one thing, appointments
usually are geared towards fixing something, and quite frankly, I
couldn't find even one thing wrong with Dean. Another was simply

how surreal it was to be brought inside the actual experience of being autistic by someone who had lived in it his whole life. Much of it was terrible to listen to, but I must admit it was fascinating as well, and has made me even more determined to help as many of these affected kids as I can. Many children have given me insight to what the world of being autistic looks like, but none has done so as eloquently as Dean.

However, the main reason I will never forget that particular appointment is because of how it ended. As they were getting ready to leave, I was compelled to ask why they had come. Dean was obviously right as rain, and yet they had driven over 1,400 miles to see me. Why? Putting his hands on his son's shoulders his father replied, "You gave us our boy. The least we could do was come and thank you face to face."

Follow-up:

According to his ND, Dean took off from there and never looked back. Since that day in November of 2011, I have not personally heard from them as there was no need for follow up. There was no actual need for them to have ever come in at all really, and it could have easily been one of the many cases where the family takes matters into their own hands, does the Protocol on their own, and heals their kids themselves, and I never even hear about them. The only reason I even knew about Dean is because of the grace and generosity of his amazing parents who drove 1,400 miles, just to say thank you.

You're very welcome.

CASE STUDY 10

Mom: *"Are you telling me that all this was caused by a cereal?"*

Does not talk yet - lots of temp/tantrums lately
Escalating very quickly
No language? (unfocused) eye contact

Name: Jenna F. (Female)

Age: 1.5
DX: None
Other diets: Breastfed. Paleo with one notable exception
No vaccines

Jenna is an interesting case for one big reason. She had none of the common factors that are generally associated with an autism risk, and yet she was definitely going down that path. She was breastfed for over a year, she had no vaccines, and she was now eating Paleo-approved foods since her whole family had been doing that for years. So what happened?

Being that she is the youngest child of a family that has been with me all thirteen years of my practice, they got her in at the first sign of trouble. It was actually her now teenaged sister, whom I've been working with since she was four, who demanded that Jenna be brought in to see me, and she was there with her mom during the appointment, monitoring the whole process.

This family actually is more like two families. They have an older boy and girl (both in their teens), then two very young children. Jenna, at one-and-a-half was an "oops" baby, and her planned brother, who was also sort of present for this appointment as he was currently residing in Mom, even younger. Working with them was always a joy since the two older kids seem to function as an extra set of parents to the little ones. Being a working mom with kids to look after, seemingly little things can easily slip through the cracks, and it was the big sister who noticed the problems sneaking into Jenna's life before anyone else did.

Looking at Jenna, it was difficult to think there could be anything "wrong" with this child. For one thing she was (and still is) one of the most beautiful children I've ever seen. Tall and strong for her young age, her dark blonde hair is set off by incredibly lovely eyes. She still teases me about it because I used to call her "Opal Eyes."

While her Mom and I were talking (with big sister chiming in, of course) I began to immediately notice the symptoms they were telling me about that were causing their concern. She would let me hold her, but she would not make any eye contact. She picked up a letter opener from my desk and immediately became fascinated with it to the exclusion of anything else going in the room. When her sister tried to take it from her, she yelled and swatted at her. Strangely, that yell was the first sound I had heard her make. She did not say, "no," or "mine;" it was just an aggrieved yelp.

Her mom confirmed that Jenna had no speech whatsoever -- no words, very few sounds, not even any baby babbling. At this stage in her development she should have had at least some speech and the lack of it was really starting to concern them. She had also recently begun having temper tantrums that were very quickly and alarmingly escalating.

Her motor skills were not developing either and she was having trouble holding anything. Spoons, forks, even larger things like crayons were all out of the question. When they asked the pediatrician about it, he had suggested that they have her eat a certain breakfast cereal off her highchair tray to improve her motor skills. "It didn't seem to help at all, and in fact, it seems kind of worse. And her tantrums are getting awful."

No wonder. They had just revealed the source of Jenna's high manganese. This cereal, recommended by "four out of five pediatricians" (according to its literature) is "fortified with vitamins and minerals," including manganese. Tons of it. With the daily suggested amount being between 2-3 mg for a full-grown adult, little bitty Jenna was getting over 3.5 mg of manganese in each 3.5 ounce serving. A massive overdose. No wonder her symptoms were escalating! By the way, a tip of the cap to that one hold-out pediatrician who doesn't recommend this cereal. You go Doctor Number Five!

When I explained Jenna's manganese overload to her mother, she couldn't believe it. Shaking her head, she said, "So let me get this straight. I did an all-natural pregnancy, breast fed for over a year, Paleo food after that with this one exception, no vaccines, and we're getting done in by a stupid breakfast cereal?" Yep, afraid so. Fortunately I had over a decade of trust with her, so she accepted it with no further questions.

It fact, she started digging around in her purse and merely said, "Trash can." I brought it out from under my desk and she unceremoniously dropped a plastic bag fully loaded with the offending morsels into the trash. Sighing again, she asked, "Alright then. How do we fix this?" I wish everyone was so compliant! We decided to start Jenna on Phase 1 of the Protocol, and I was confident she would begin that very day. Not to mention that the source of Jenna's issues was already residing in the trash under my desk.

<u>One-month progress report:</u>

As I had expected, Phase 1 had gone into full swing the first day, and Jenna's swift progress was reflecting their diligence. Within a week, Jenna had not only started to talk with "new words every day," she was now spending most of the day happily singing. Instead of the hyper-focus she had been showing, she was now playing, laughing and singing all day while she went from one project to another with the rest of the gang.

While the teenaged kids were working on a jigsaw puzzle one night, Jenna's previously nonexistent motor skills suddenly kicked in, and she was easily able to help find and fit in puzzle pieces. They had bought her some less complex puzzles of her own that are designed for younger children, and she was enjoying doing them by herself, but she still liked to get involved with the older siblings.

As it so often happens, the minute her speech kicked in, the tantrums stopped. Since she could now tell people what she wanted, and maybe more importantly being that she had brothers and sisters, what she didn't want, her frustration level had abated.

She was starting to form her own opinions about what she wanted to wear and what she wanted to do, but there was one thing she was absolutely adamant about. The diapers had to go. When her mom got busy and forgot they were working on potty training, Jenna actually took care of business by herself.

As I stated before, this family has been seeing me for many years and so are quite knowledgeable about natural medicine. Thinking that her spirulina could help speed up the iron-loading process, her mom handed her a capsule of it one morning while taking her own supplements. From that day on, Jenna became one of my many "spirulina chewers!"

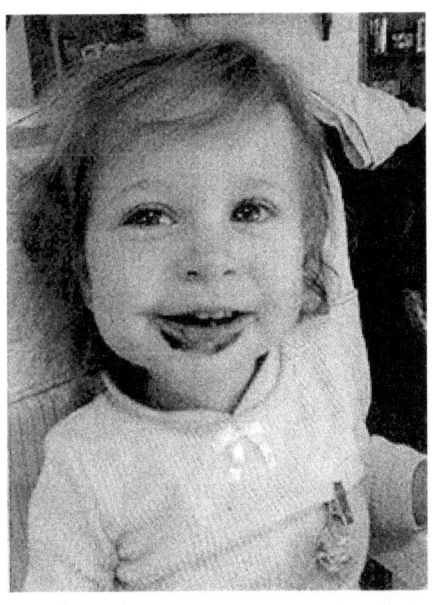

If you've never tasted spirulina, I will tell you that in my mind it tastes exactly like what it is; pond scum. Okay, technically it is a blue-green freshwater algae, and it is exceedingly good for you, but *blech*! Not a good flavor! It just goes to show you that kids often instinctively know what is good for them because Jenna is only one in a long line of kids who actually like to chew the capsules up. I have the cutest picture of her in a baby chair laughing with the green spirulina totally festooning her face! I'm glad I didn't have to clean up *that* one.

Jenna was obviously doing great, so I suggested that they go on to Phase 2 of the Protocol and we'd do a check in with her next month, just to be certain.

Two-month progress report:

Ever since I wrote my first book ("If Naturopaths Are Quacks, Then I Guess I'm A Duck"), clients have been giving me gifts of rubber duckies. I currently have over three hundred of them from all over the world. One of them, a blue one from Germany, happened to be sitting on my desk when they came in for the appointment. Jenna ran in and excitedly picked it up. Holding it up to me, she asked, "You know what ducks say, Dr. Shauna? Quack, quack, quack!"

As she went around my office looking at some of the other ducks, and quacking at them as well, I observed, "It looks like we're good here." Nodding her head, Mom agreed. "Nothing to see here. Move along," she joked.

And there was nothing. Jenna had gone from silence and temper tantrums to complete sentences and a happy little girl calmness. She was loving her puzzles, although they had needed to kick the simplicity level up a few notches, and she was developing an avid interest in books. Her language skills were now far exceeding "age appropriate" and were quickly making the transition to "advanced". She was gaining a lot of independence and was very proud to tell me about her new "big girl bed" she had received as a present this month.

As she continued to walk around naming all my ducks, Mom shook her head. "It's so amazing, this whole thing. It was so easy and so fast. Amazing." Her older daughter seemed perplexed by that statement. Giving me a quizzical look she asked "Why is it amazing? Isn't this how it's supposed to work?" That kid. Always my fan. Even miracles don't faze her.

Follow-up:

This case was a clear and powerful lesson on how easily the iron/manganese imbalance can be upset in kids, especially very young ones. The family was doing everything right except one seemingly tiny thing. Who could imagine that a cereal could cause such a train wreck in a child's life? The "a little bit won't hurt" attitude that drives me so crazy? It's wrong. Just remember: Even "a little bit" of something off the Protocol-approved foods can keep it from working at all. It's not worth it.

Since the entire family follows a Paleo diet, there have never been any more issues with Jenna. She's five now and I see her from time to time for other unrelated issues, or when another family member comes in. Just like the rest of the kids in this family, she is extremely intelligent, sweet, beautiful and all around an exceptional child. And she still looks straight at me with those amazing opal eyes.

CHAPTER SIX

The Spectrum Balance® Protocol

The primary focus in current autism research has shifted dramatically in course in the last few years from trying to help the children who are already affected in some way, to now prevention before it happens. While this is well and good, what about the vast numbers of children (and children becoming adults) who are already affected? It seems that they are being mostly medicated and mitigated as opposed to helped.

The role of the Spectrum Balance® Protocol is to reverse this damage that has been caused by a simple mineral imbalance. It has to start by increasing iron absorption and bio-availability. **Even if there is plenty of iron in your food, or if you're taking supplements, it doesn't matter if it isn't bio-available.**

Again, a Band-Aid approach of taking an iron supplement is not going to fix the issue. As long as you are eating grains and other phytate-containing foods, iron and other needed minerals in your body will continue to be chelated, or washed out. I've seen kids on massive amounts of supplements and yet their tests still show a near depletion of the very vitamins and minerals they are taking. The parents are then told that their child is a "slow absorber" or one of the many other terms that have been coined, when in fact, the reason they can't hold onto their minerals is because of the phytates in the grains and cereals they're eating for breakfast, or their sandwich for lunch!

Of course, prevention is key, and as you can see by using this Protocol while pregnant and in your child's early life, it is easily doable. But what about all the people who are already affected? Do we just give up and "accept them the way they are"? Throw the baby out with the bathwater?

No!

What the Spectrum Balance® Protocol has proved in its (thus far) nine years of use is that even though the damage has already occurred, even if it was a long time ago, it can, through the targeted use of real food, be reduced or many times reversed. The idea that there is nothing you can do, that there is no hope...is simply not true.

One thing to keep in mind is to not over-complicate this Protocol. Strangely enough, one of the largest stumbling blocks I have found is that it often seems too simple a solution to feel real to many parents. Although it is difficult to believe that so many symptoms could possibly be caused by something so basic, that's what we've discovered to be true. As a result, the Protocol is often perceived as "too easy," especially for those who have been engaging in complicated and expensive biomedical testing and treatments.

The prevailing mindset held by a majority of Americans is that the only way to successfully tackle any disease is through drugs, surgery or other expensive and invasive treatments. While these absolutely have their places in restoring health and fixing damaged or ill organs or systems, I firmly believe that utilizing a dietary approach first, especially when it comes to ever more pervasive conditions such as autism only makes sense. Currently, various research and charity groups that are, by their own admission, "desperately seeking answers" for autism are not yet even seriously considering the link between diet and symptoms expressed in ASDs. Perhaps this is because it is often the nature of highly educated and intelligent people (like physicians and researchers) to seek complexity when sometimes, something as simple as diet modification may be that correct solution. The truth is that many of the very best things in life are simple, so please don't allow this subversive mindset to keep you from trying this Protocol with your children!

Stop and think about this for a minute. It has only been since the explosion of packaged, grain-based, and convenience foods that we have had a concomitant rise of autism and autism spectrum disorders. Think back to your own formative years. How many "special needs" kids went to your school? I myself went to a massive elementary school in Southern California in the late 1960's/early 1970's and yet there were no autistic children in the Special Ed classes. It has to be our diet. It's the only thing that makes sense!

The best news about using the Spectrum Balance® Protocol is that once the manganese and iron are restored into proper, healthy balance in the brain, it stays that way unless you throw it off again, which is not all that easy to do. Granted, since I will never meet the mass majority of the people using this in the 67 countries it's it has been downloaded in thus far, there could be some circumstances that I am not aware of. However, I will tell you that the only reversals that occur after that balance has been achieved and that I have personally witnessed have been from one cause. Grains! And once they took the grains out again they were able to regain their lost ground.

The most common question I hear is, "What is your typical result?" As if people can be typical! I will say that in general the ones who eat from my "best" list of foods the most, those who have less time affected, and the people with less body weight - especially little kids - have the fastest result, which only makes sense. However, the "general rule" is that we see at least some positive forward motion in the first few weeks. I always suggest that people give it a minimum of 90 days, but we usually see enough positive changes within that time period to keep them going without much additional urging.

The question of the children who are on medication is an FAQ as well. Since the drugs have a tendency to mask symptoms it is sometimes harder to discern if they are making progress, and drugs often do have a marked tendency to slow the progress. However, with the mass majority of kids I've worked with who were on medications, we still saw great results. It just takes a little longer and you need to watch them more closely for signs of positive forward motion.

Keep in mind that sometimes the "positive forward motion" doesn't appear on the surface to be positive. Although it is the mass exception and not the rule, I have seen some children whose symptoms ramped up significantly before subsiding. They will also sometimes exhibit very positive changes for six to eight weeks, then have a complete blow out for a few days before continuing on their forward path. I asked my friend Joe Dispenza, who is one of the world's experts on neurotransmitters, what he in his expert opinion thought about why this would occur. He laughed at me and said, "Because change is hard!" All too true -- and back to that idea of simplicity.

One of the strangest examples of this was a child who made steady progress for about four weeks, then had what appeared to be a stomach flu and vomited for nearly 24 hours straight. The next morning he began speaking words for the first time. We thought it was coincidental until he did it again four weeks later, and the day after his "flu" he woke up speaking in sentences. He continued this pattern several more times until he reached final balance. I've never seen anything like it before or since and truthfully I have no explanation for it. Getting back to the idea that there's no such thing as "typical" when it comes to the human body. Whatever it was it worked, so I'll take it!

Some families have only had to strictly adhere to the Protocol for as short a time period as three to six months, while others have shown steady improvement during the course of years. A few have chosen to stay on it indefinitely. When your six-year-old was ramming his head through the drywall and threatening to kill himself and others despite his anti-psychotic meds, I think you have more of a tendency to say "If it ain't broke..." and stay on it indefinitely. This is not a problem of course, as the Spectrum Balance® Protocol is a very sustainable and healthy form of a Paleo diet.

And the big question on everyone's mind? "When is it time to get off it?" Answer: When your child is right where you want him or her to be! We've proven over and over that numbers on tests are a lot less important than the behavior and health of your child. What I care about is results! So when they both you and your child are perfectly happy with how they behave and feel, then you're done.

We all know the truth on this. If you want to be truly healthy, you can't go back to eating your "old" diet, which is most likely what landed you here in the first place. It's the same for dietary changes to achieve weight loss; once you hit your goal weight if you revert back to the bad stuff, the weight reappears. It's not rocket science. As for the kids, think of it this way -- if you stuck your hand in a beehive and got stung, would you do it again? Likely not. And neither would your child want to eat something that they know through experience ruins their day! Their cravings for unhealthy foods will fade away as long as healthy foods stay in the house, the disallowed ones stay out, and as long as your attitude about healthy food stays positive. Kids learn best by your example, not your words. So be a good example!

Junk food and grains and the like will never be good for you. But isn't it nice to think that being off your regular diet occasionally is at least not going to result in a catastrophe? As soon as the imbalance is corrected it will most likely stay that way unless too many grains start sneaking back into their diet. Once your child's healthy iron-manganese balance is restored if they happen to consume some "bad" food here and there, the result is more likely to be a tummy ache than a melt-down. Won't that be a nice change?

11 - 15

In any dietary protocol, it seems that "cheating" on your diet will eventually become a topic of discussion. I personally don't like the term "cheating", since you really aren't cheating on anyone but yourself, but it is the prevalent nomenclature.

If you look at support groups, especially on social media, "cheating" is not looked at as any big thing, and the standard advice is to pick yourself up, dust yourself off, and get back on the wagon. If you are dieting to lose weight or otherwise gain self-improvement, this advice is probably reasonable. **However, if you are on the Spectrum Balance Protocol the advice is completely counterproductive.**

I know I'm repeating myself, but always remember that **90% (or sometimes even 99%) compliance to this Protocol will usually yield 0% results!**

Some advice that I often give my clients about "cheats", is to "Use the right word" when thinking about it. Any foods that are on the "avoid" list of the Spectrum Balance® Protocol are currently going to be a disaster to your child. Many will return to being healthy after the iron and manganese balance is corrected, but for now they are potential minefields to your success. So use the "Right word". Poison. Instead of saying "Oh one little cookie can't hurt", say "Oh one little dose of poison can't hurt". Yowch. Sounds a lot different that way doesn't it? Makes it much easier to stay away from...

In case you still think that "a little bit can't hurt anything" the following case studies will change your mind. Who knew that a pineapple could turn a five-year-old boy into a Tasmanian Devil?

CASE STUDY 11

Mom: *"This is so amazing!"*

Ax: S
Comments: What questions can I ask you
on the phone that will let us see
if he is better?

Notes:
1. Speaks a lot - vy loud
2. Laughs hard at notley- "Constantly giggling"
3. Looks like his usual self... tc.

Name: Cole F. (Male)

Age: 5
DX: Autism
Other diets: GFCF, GAPS
RX: Nyastatin several times for yeast. None current.
ND: Cyndi Ringoen

Cole is yet another in the string of successful outcomes we had without me ever actually meeting him in person but all through phone consultations. It is important to remember that this Protocol can and has worked many many times with no practitioner supervision, which is why this book can be so effectively used. He also proves once again what a dynamite combo it is when you combine the Spectrum Balance Protocol and neurodevelopmental work!

At age two, Cole's parents started to notice that things were not quite right with their son. He had no speech at all and was flapping his arms almost constantly (his "stim"). The term "stimming" is short for self-stimulatory behavior, sometimes also called "stereotypic" behavior. In a person with autism, stimming usually refers to these specific behaviors which may include flapping, rocking, spinning, or repetition of words and phrases.

Stimming is one of the most common and easily recognizable symptoms of autism, but it's important to note that stimming is also a part of most people's behavior patterns. Most people "stim" as a way to calm themselves or as a nervous habit of sorts. If you've ever tapped your pencil, bitten your nails, twirled your hair, or paced when you're nervous, then you've engaged in stimming.

Since Cole has apraxia, his parents felt that it might be just that arresting his speech, but when he started walking around the house tracing all the walls (known as "wall walking," it is a common symptom of autism) they took him to his pediatrician. After some testing, the doctor noted that his manganese level was "off the charts" but assured them that this was "no problem." As they suspected, he was diagnosed with autism shortly after that at age two-and-a-half.

Wanting to do the best for their son, they immediately began working with an autism specialist. Under his direction they did yeast detoxes, supplement programs, ABA therapy as well as the GFCF and GAPS diets. Despite all of those programs and treatments, at age five Cole was still stuck at a developmental age of three.

Luckily for Cole his parents had not given up on him, and his mom's internet research led her to a neurodevelopmentalist I work with who was in their area. Immediately, Cyndi suggested that they start my Protocol, as she does with all her clients. Since the family had already been through so many diets and programs, they were pretty worn out by all this trial-and-error, and didn't have much faith in trying yet another. After reviewing my Protocol, they decided that it was "too much work" as they had already been on so many specialized diets with no significant result. Because of this "diet burnout," I can't really blame them for not having the steam to go ahead.

Fortunately for him his ND kept the pressure on, and after her strong-arming them for several months they decided to take the plunge; although by their own admission their approach to the Protocol was more like putting a toe in the water than a "plunge." While I always suggest that everyone should start as strictly as possible on Phase 1, they were eating a fairly loose Phase 2 diet. Although starting with Phase 2 is far from optimal and therefore cuts down the chance of seeing any dramatic change, Cole was fortunate and they saw many positives anyway. In approximately two weeks his life-long diarrhea had stopped, he was sleeping better, he was flapping and stimming less, and most significantly, "he looks like he wants to talk."

Even with his progress moving forward so rapidly, his parents remained unconvinced that it was the diet that was causing the positive changes. It seemed like too much change too quickly for it to be just the dietary change. Based on this mindset, they decided that it wouldn't hurt anything to start adding "snacks" back into his diet. Almost immediately (and predictably) "he went straight back to square one." Okay, more convinced now! This was enough proof for Mom to make an appointment for a phone consultation with me, so she could get "the most benefit" from having Cole on the Protocol.

It is very important so I will mention again that Cole got lucky here. Nine times out of ten if you start on anything other than Phase 1 you won't see much if any recognizable change, especially in such a short period of time. I have heard this same story from dozens of people who tried to start on Phase 2 because it was easier and closer to what they were already eating, and got little or no result. Then at a later time on the advice of their ND, friend, doctor, or arm-twisting family member, decided to go full force on to Phase 1 only to see the same quick results that occurred in Cole and so many others. I'm not exactly sure why it happened this way for him. My best hypothesis is that because he had been on the gut-healing diets of both GFCF and GAPS in the past, the only issue left to address was the manganese imbalance, so it jumpstarted. **For the record, I do not recommend that anyone ever start on anything other than Phase 1.**

Although Cole had a lot of what most would call classic autism symptoms, he also had a few that I considered to be iffy. It is sometimes necessary to sort through what the symptoms of autism are and what are merely little kid behaviors. His main symptoms of no speech, having difficulty crossing thresholds (because it represents too much change), having "fits" where he didn't seem to know where he was or what he was doing, not being potty trained, and flapping all fit in with autism. A few, like his "laughing at nothing" his mom spoke of just seemed like a kid behavior to me, since I see "normal" kids do that all the time. In most cases when I hear this type of behavior relayed as a symptom, it is generally coming from someone who expects the house to be quieter than it is with a five-year-old in it.

One I could agree with was the high-pitched squeals that he regularly emitted. I don't know if you've ever heard one of these "stim" squeals, but it not only tortures your ears, it seems to reverberate through your whole body. Even just hearing him in the background while I was on the phone with his mom was enough to make me agree that had to stop!

Since she was already familiar with the Protocol, most of what I did with her during our consultation was to stress the importance of being as strict as possible on Phase 1, and to forgo any usual "snacks." As happens quite often, she informed me that Dad would not be joining them on the Protocol, and she was concerned that Cole would get into his snacks. I stressed that it is optimal to get everyone on the diet together, but no matter what she had to get all forbidden food out of the house. She was dubious on this point, but said she'd do her best.

One-month progress report: (phone)

Although Mom had done what she could about getting all the contraband food out of the house, she had unfortunately been overridden. As a result, Cole would do very well on the diet for awhile, but would have inexplicable regressions from time to time. The basis of these regressions were fully explained one night when they turned on the lights and caught five-year-old Cole climbing the kitchen cabinets up to his Dad's hidden stash, which they didn't even know he knew was up there. I don't know how the kids know but they always do, and this is far from the only kid I've heard of that has climbed furniture or cabinets, or even picked locks, to get to some off-Protocol goodies. After that the forbidden cabinet was cleaned out, dad ate his snacks outside the house, and the regressions predictably stopped.

Now that he was purely on Phase 1, Cole was hitting his stride. The "fits" and the flapping simply stopped over the course of a few short weeks, and he rarely even seemed to notice thresholds anymore. His speech, completely nonexistent only a month prior, was now bubbling out of him. "Not only is he talking but he's connecting words when he's worked with. He has apraxia, which makes it more difficult to understand him, but he's trying so hard."

Putting his new language skills to work, Cole had started asking for sausage and eggs for breakfast, and reminding his mom about what foods he wanted when they were at the grocery store. He was starting to have his own mind and opinions and was making a lot of his own choices -- not only about what he wanted to eat, but about which clothes he wanted to wear, and which of his toys he wanted to play with. "He has an opinion now. It's awesome!" Mom enthused.

Thankfully, the incidences of his squealing had gone down to the point that he only did it when he was excited, which was making everyone happier. What hadn't stopped was his "laughing at nothing" behavior, and she was pretty concerned about it. I again explained, that in my opinion, I did not think that was an autistic behavior, and I wasn't sure if she could expect that one to change. I could tell by her lackluster response that she was not thrilled with that particular opinion of mine.

<u>Two-month progress report: (phone)</u>

It has long been my custom in my practice to take free phone calls from nine to ten in the morning when anyone, whether a client or not, can call in and ask questions. Since this report was not a formally scheduled one, just one of those ten-minute calls during that time, it is a bit more brief.

Cole was doing great! None of the original symptoms of the "fits" or flapping had reoccurred and the "too much change" issue that kept him from crossing thresholds had stayed out of his life as well. Although his speech was still more difficult to understand because of the apraxia, he was having no problems getting his points across and was doing fantastic in school. "He knows what he's saying and follows directions really well. His communicating is awesome."

When a kid is doing this great, it's usually when I ask the question, "So what do we have left to do?" Answer: "The giggles. He giggles for no reason." Really? Again? My response was, "Look, he's just a happy little five-year-old. Maybe stuff is funny to him that you just don't get because you're not five. I really think you're stuck with that one until he grows out of it. Could be worse, right?" Apparently they still weren't crazy about the giggles. I guess since I never saw it happen it could have been worse than I thought, but it seemed better to me than flapping and fits of anger. Her response to his giggling continued to mystify me.

Progress report: (phone)

The next communication took place over four months later, during which "the holidays" had occurred, and again, was just a brief 9am phone call. The Holidays. Sigh. Don't get me wrong, I love Halloween, Thanksgiving and Christmas as much as anyone, but in my line of work you come to dread them as a black hole where good diets go to die.

Mom's first comment wasn't unexpected. "We weren't super strict over the holidays and he got horrible." That will happen. Especially when eating what most people think of as "holiday food." Since Cole's Protocol diet had never been what I consider "super strict", the iron and manganese imbalance had stayed... well... imbalanced, and it was therefore easier for him to regress. It is very important that this balance gets achieved and stabilized prior to eating any of the "avoid" foods, or chances are you'll be thrown right back off again. Once it is established, a little off-the-diet-food doesn't do

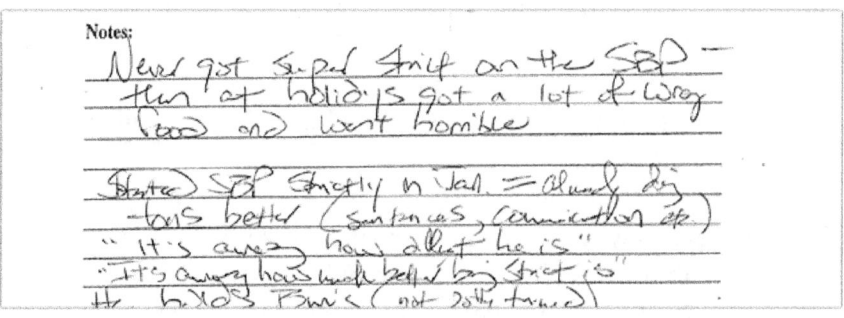

much, although most do stay a bit more sensitive to high manganese foods or supplements. It is especially challenging when it's the time of year when candy, sugar, bread and desserts seem to become their own food groups.

My suggestion was that they do a reboot. Go back to square one for a bit and see what happens. Mom agreed to go back to Phase 1, and would let me know how it went.

One-month later: (phone)

"It's amazing how much better he is when we're being strict," Cole's mom declared.

Within one month of being strictly on Phase 1, we were back in business. All of Cole's newly acquired skills of forming sentences, communication and co-operation kicked right back in as if he'd never lost them. Although it's not uncommon for people to fall off the wagon (especially around the holidays), I've always been glad to see that once a child has been on track, it's not too difficult to get right back on again when they fall off. Although the child may regress for a bit, if you don't let it get too far out of control, we can usually get them back pretty quickly.

Cole's gains in his communication skills were getting better by the day, and had made more new strides in the last month. "He's stringing words together like crazy. He yells sometimes but at least he has an opinion. It's awesome." Awesome! Mom's favorite adjective always made me smile.

What was very new (and no less awesome) was that he was starting to interact with other children, and had his very first "real conversation" *ever in his life* the day before this appointment. Starting out at a developmental age of only three, Cole's world was opening up his now five-year-old mind. He was becoming interested in the outside world; watching TV, asking questions about other people, and especially wanting to go to Little League games. He was becoming extremely self-aware and was realizing that he could and should defend himself. Mom gave an example: "His sister took a toy, which she's always been able to do without him noticing, and he said, 'That's not yours, give it!' This has been so amazing." (I'll take that "a" word, too!)

Cole's ND, his mom, and I, were all in agreement that the only thing left now was for him to have some time to catch up. What a journey for a kid to go from being three to being five in just a few short months! He had a few old habits to release, and some new ones to gain, but other than that, he was good to go.

Oh. Except the giggling. He was still giggling.

Follow-up:

I last spoke to Cole's mother in February of 2012. Both she and Cole's ND reported that he was catching up quickly, and was doing great. The family made the decision to stay on the Phase 3 part of the Protocol, as they found it to be very easily maintainable and he was doing very well on it. Although he had eaten a few "avoid" foods over the holidays (of course) this year, they had not caused any negative effect.

This is probably as good a place as any to mention that I've been told that I can be a bit tough. I can live with that. I'm not here to be a buddy, I'm here to get your kids well, and a lot fewer of them would have recovered if I wasn't "tough" at times. Usually, people wind up thanking me for it, but not everyone. Cole's mom was one that thought that I was pretty tough, but I think that was only because of the one niggling issue we continued to disagree on.

He was still giggling. His mom remained a bit irritated with me that I didn't consider that to be autistic behavior, but I stuck to my guns on this one. My goal is for the kids to be happy and healthy, and free from the sensory overload issues, nightmares, anxiety and other Menefe Syndrome related issues. It is NOT my goal that they lose their personalities in any way, or stop acting like kids. In my opinion, kids should be allowed to act like kids. Kids giggle.

Since it's now almost three years later, maybe they've worked out that giggling issue. Or not. Seems pretty much up to Cole!

CASE STUDY 12

Mom: *"He's a totally different child."*

> Mostly behavioral problems =
> In a group of kids he will not interact
> Does not like to be restrained in any way
> When he is outside he's fine but if you
> try to bring him in "he has a meltdown"
> Wants to sleep with parents, bad dreams
> often –

Name: Zack B. (Male)

Age: 4
DX: None officially
Other diets: None

Since I practice on the sunny southern border of Colorado and New Mexico it's not unusual to see people come in wearing sunglasses, and a few who will keep them on inside if they're only in briefly. It is unusual to have a four-year-old wear them for the entire one hour appointment, but Zack just couldn't take that much sunlight. Clue number one.

Zack and his parents had been referred in by a dear friend of mine because, like many I see, they just didn't know where else to turn. It takes a lot to pack your child into a car and drive for over 1,000 miles each way under any circumstances, but they had done it with Zack yelling his head off most of the way.

They knew that there were severe and escalating problems with him, but like many families they didn't want to get him in an official "loop," so they had avoided getting a diagnosis. As I am writing this, the official number for an autism diagnosis in boys is thought to be 1 in 54, yet here was another boy who was so obviously was on the ASD spectrum and who was not diagnosed, like so many I see. I often wonder, what is the real number?

If you had told me during that first appointment that Zack would become one of my favorite clients, it would have been a very hard sell. He had not one, but two, screaming melt-downs in less than an hour, and being that I am blessed (cursed?) with very delicate hearing it was quite the trial. It did however, show me up close and personal what kind of situation his parents were dealing with.

Apparently, these tantrums were all too common. Mom explained, "If he's outside and we want him to come in, he has a melt-down. If he's inside and we want him to come out, he has a melt-down. It's pretty much about anything." The entire family was being controlled by his behavior as it was impossible to guess where or when he would launch into one of these fits.

For those of you who don't have a child who has "melt-downs" or has ever witnessed one, let me explain the difference. "Normal" kids (for lack of a better term) who throw tantrums can be generally calmed down and reasoned with, and they usually have an identifiable "trigger," such as having to go to school, a doctor's appointment, or not getting a toy they want at the store. Usually they will calm down with either discipline and/or the promise of a later reward. When a child "melts-down" there is no way to reason with them, and it is doubtful if the child can even hear you. It is not uncommon for the child, a parent, or a sibling to be physically injured during one of these episodes. Speaking for myself, some pieces of my office furniture have been the unfortunate victims of melt downs, but my body primarily escaped too much damage. The worst part is that unlike with other kids, there is rarely any identifiable trigger, so there is nothing you know you need to avoid in public or in social situations. They just go off to the races and you never know where or when it will happen or how long it will last. It's a real nightmare for the families.

As severe as Zack's melt-downs were, and they were their top concern, he had a host of other issues. Due to start kindergarten in a few months, it was apparent that it would be impossible to do so in his present situation. Despite the additional "special education" classes he was currently in to get prepared for it, he was nowhere near ready to be in school. He had no focus whatsoever and his speech, garbled and slow, was nearly impossible to understand. His social interaction with other kids was described by the teachers in one word: Zero. This was in June 2008, and he was supposed to start school in September. It wasn't looking good.

Before the first melt-down he had in my office, Zack was acting very tired and cranky. I was willing to give him the benefit of the doubt after his long car ride, but it turned out that they had actually arrived two days earlier and had been staying with my friend who had referred them. His mom told me that he was rarely rested and attributed that to the screaming nightmares that drove him into his parents bed nearly every night. "I can hardly remember the last time my husband and I have slept alone," she sighed.

When we got down to discussing the actual Protocol, we hit our first speed bump. They were eating what I would classify as a fairly typical Southern diet. I was introduced to this when I lived in Nashville, so I knew what to expect. Biscuits and gravy, pancakes or cereal for breakfast, sandwiches mostly for lunch, and something breaded for dinner. Grains, grains and more grains.

As much as she wanted to try the Protocol, Mom simply couldn't get her mind wrapped around the idea of changing their diet nearly

100%. "What do you eat for breakfast on this thing, for heaven's sake?" As we discussed recipe ideas, and especially when I encouraged her to keep things very simple (bacon and eggs, just no toast), she started to calm down. She's not the first person I've had to peel off the ceiling when they first see the diet! People who are used to eating "cultural diets" of some sort are nearly always the hardest ones to encourage to make this change. It seems that every area of the country (and the world for that matter) has its own food habits and preferences and some are harder to change than others. I even had one woman who told me that it was "impossible for people from Wisconsin to eat like this." I beg to differ.

Even though Mom was much calmer by the end of the appointment, this was another of those cases that probably would have never happened had it not been for the strong recommendation from my friend, her cousin. That, and the fact that there weren't a lot of options left for Zack. The Protocol was once again, as I've heard so many times, their last resort.

One-month progress report: (Phone)

As predicted, the family had a bit of a hard time getting started on the Protocol. The house was chock full of no-no's and they were in a life-long pattern of cooking a certain way. Mom and Dad had to have a few serious sit downs to figure out what new foods they could eat and find some new recipes to replace the old. Thank goodness for all the wonderful Paleo foods websites there are out there to help! They found many recipes on those sites that only had to be minimally altered that they felt could work for them.

It took a few weeks to really get going, but once they did... bang! Zack began to change almost as soon as he started the Protocol. Mom witnessed a whole series of very big changes that had taken place in just the first few weeks.

Zack's behavior had taken a sharp, positive U-turn. As Mom described, "For the most part, he's just a normal four-year-old boy. It's crazy." The melt-downs, although still there a bit, were not as frequent or as severe. "If he starts one we can talk him out of it now."

His speech emerged very quickly and was already much more complex and intelligible. The speech therapist he had been working with described his progress as "like magic." They were getting ready to do another evaluation before school started on him to see if he even still needed the extra help.

The nightmares were disappearing as fast as his other symptoms, which I'm sure was a relief to everyone, especially Zack. "He's sleeping in his own bed at least 90% of the time now, so we're all getting some sleep."

Once Mom had found her sea legs with the Protocol, she was feeling more confident. It was at this point that I warned her about putting in too many "goodies" and how disastrous that can be to the efficacy of the Protocol. Just like any Paleo diet, you want the focus to be on real whole foods and not on how to transform cookies, pies, and cakes into "Paleo" -- real foods will always need to be your "go to" first choice. I advised her, as I do everyone, to leave treats for special occasions only. She admitted that it was some advice she needed to hear. "We do love our pies!" she laughed.

Four-days later: (email)

To those who continue to think that "a little bit can't hurt," I give you...The Pineapple Incident.

(Email): *"I have to tell you about this incident. We've been very careful on the diet and have had some slips here and there, but this one was a doozy! Wow!"*

went off the one I made. (should have compared the list, but hindsight is 20/20) Anyway, before we talked this morning, I gave ▓▓▓ pineapple with his cereal (puffed brown rice), as pineapple was an allowed food from the blood type book. ANYWAY, that is why I was a bit surprised when you said no, he couldn't eat it! Of course it was there on your list in black and white!! DUH!! I've got to tell you, we went to town early this afternoon and it was like starting from square one!! He was in major confusion. He did not know what he wanted to do. He dropped a coin on the floor in the store and was sooooooo upset, I thought I was going to have to walk out, then he didn't want me to push the cart, he didn't want to push the cart, he didn't really know what to do, it was AMAZING to see him like this!!! I knew it was the pineapple causing this. This was the only time he's had pineapple (and last) and it is amazing the change that made!! He is doing better now, as I gave him some yogurt and raisins and some time has passed. Wow, it scared me to think how he was and how we had delt with this for so long! He's come such a long way and it brings tears of happiness that we won't have to go thru this anymore!! Thank you!!!!!

Still being new to the diet, Mom accidentally gave Zack some pineapple for breakfast. Although normally a healthy fruit, pineapple is on the avoid list because of its very high manganese content. And it showed.

Going into town with his mother to grocery shop that afternoon, Zack "went back to square one." In the store he was suddenly very confused. He didn't want to push the cart, then got mad at his mom when she did. He dropped a coin on the floor and very nearly went into a melt-down looking for it. As he had not acted this way in a long time, his mom started looking for the trigger.

(Email): *"This was the only time he's had pineapple (and the last) and it is amazing the changes that made!"*

Fortunately, it didn't do any permanent damage to his progress, and Zack was back to normal the next day. The upside to this is that it did bring home to his family how important it is to be diligent on the Protocol, and showed what disastrous effects manganese has on Zack! It was a big lesson demonstrating the importance of not cheating.

She signed off her email with: *"Wow. It scared me to think how he was and how we dealt with it for so long! It brings tears of happiness that we won't have to go through this anymore! Thank you!"*

Two-month progress report: (phone)

This month, due to some new encouraging test results and mutual agreement all around, Zack had been taken out of all his "special needs" programs, and he had begun kindergarten on schedule. His new teacher was very pleased with him, commenting that he was well behaved, learning reading and writing very quickly, and took his naps when he was supposed to. "The only odd thing is he doesn't want anyone touching his lunch." Ha! Smart kid -- he knew what was making him feel better and he was going to protect it!

In two months his behavior was now very nearly 180 degrees from where we started. His melt-downs were completely gone, and he was becoming very social at school. A recent trip to Grandma's house caused her to cease her criticism of the family being "on that weird diet" (how can a child not eat biscuits?) as she pronounced him "a totally different child."

Zack's speech had advanced even more, and he was now always speaking without hesitation in full sentences. His pace of speaking was up to normal; he was completely intelligible and expressing himself very well.

Since the holidays were coming up (gulp) and we wouldn't be talking for awhile due to their travel schedule, I gave Mom all the usual warnings about holiday food and too many snacks, and re-minded her of The Pineapple Incident. As if I needed to. I think that particular occurrence was burned into her consciousness.

When I asked if there were any issues to work on, she said "He's just amazing. We can go anywhere now. He's just a regular four-year-old boy." Taking that as a no, I suggested that she check in with me after the holidays to make sure he remained on the great track he was currently on.

<u>Three months later (Five months on the SBP): (phone)</u>

With all the holiday trips to the various grandparents, cousins and friends, staying on the Protocol had been a challenge, but they succeeded. Zack was still doing great! He was so confident with his speech now that he had participated in bus trips with a group of other children to perform Christmas caroling at some area nursing homes, and he had performed a speaking and singing part in the school Christmas play. Not half bad for a kid who could barely speak the previous summer!

There had been no melt-downs or other difficult behavior for so many months now that his mom said she could "barely remember them." All of his test scores were above average and his math scores were "advanced." How advanced? The math test criteria necessitated a score of 109 or more for the most advanced category, and Zack's score was 172! He was having a little trouble with his attention span in class, but my suspicion is that the classwork wasn't challenging enough for him anymore. I've seen this happen quite often as the formerly slower kids start racing past their counterparts. It's not a lack of focus, it's boredom.

When I asked if there was anything more to work on, Mom said that they were very happy with where he is now. "He's so witty and funny. He's just a happy kid."

Because Zack had already dramatically demonstrated his intolerance to manganese with The Pineapple Incident, I suggested that they stay with Phase 3 of the Protocol, and to stay away from pineapple! Mom had no trouble agreeing to that one! He was discharged in January of 2009.

Follow-up:

I got a phone call two months later from Zack's Dad, with whom I had never previously spoken. When I asked if everything was okay, he said, "Things are great. He's so smart it would blow your mind. His grades are insanely good."

The reason he called was because he felt that although Zack was flying, his wife was still being a bit over protective. He and all of Zack's teachers were thinking that he was "extremely advanced" at this point, but Mom wanted to keep him in kindergarten for another year. I let him know that this is far from unusual and that I in fact see it all the time. It's hard to let go and be less protective some-times when you've had to virtually hover over a child their entire life. It seems like it should be an easy thing to accept that your child has made enough advancements to keep up with their classmates, or in Zack's case, surpassed their classmates, but many times it's not. Since the person who referred this family in is a good friend of mine and his wife's cousin, I asked his permission to talk to her. He thought that was great and wholeheartedly seconded the idea!

When I spoke with my friend, she was point blank about it. "She's just like that. Don't worry, I'll handle it," she promised. Apparently, they had a very productive talk, because the pressure to hold Zack back slacked off immediately.

Nine months later I received an email. It was a picture of Zack showing his very own goat at a 4H event. His Mom wrote: *"He did showmanship at the county fair with his goat. He did AWESOME! I was never able to stay at the fair to watch my other son show his an-imals (because Zack always threw a fit), but Zack is SHOWING now! Doesn't he look sooooo happy?"*

Yes, he does. He's smiling, I'm smiling, and I think there is a good possibility that the goat is smiling. I love this picture.

CASE STUDY 13

Comments: Rx: none
DX: Autism (age 4 in April)
Age 4

(tried Ritalin
& Trazadone
...Ritalin medicine
a psycho)

Notes:

Name: Paul F. (Male)

Age: 4
DX: Autism
Other diets: None
RX: Had tried both Ritalin and Trazadone. "Ritalin made him a psycho."

Life did not start out well for Paul. Born to a drug-addicted mother, he didn't get his first break until his new mom took him into foster care at seven weeks old, then adopted him at age two. It is heart-breaking to see these poor kids, and I've seen many of them, who nearly automatically have health challenges through no fault of their own. I must admit that it does make it even more rewarding when we're able to bring them back to health, as we did with Paul.

One can never know absolutely for sure where a child's high manganese level could have come from, but in Paul's case, it could very easily be assumed that it was from his baby formula. I do not and will never understand why nearly all baby formulas and baby foods are so high in manganese content. Hopefully, growing the awareness about Menefe Syndrome will go a long way toward changing that! As for right now, they're loaded.

It was easy to see at first glance that this poor little guy was not happy in his body. He was like a perpetual motion machine; he couldn't sit still for a second, was constantly moving, standing up and sitting down, and seemingly unable to make eye contact. Usually I can derive some recognition from the kids if I really work at it but not this time. He was far too busy wriggling and fidgeting to be able to focus even for a few seconds. As you'd expect, kids often act differently in my office than they do at home, but according to his mom this was a constant thing. Poor guy couldn't even calm down to go to bed, and as a result, had very poor sleep patterns and was often tired.

In addition to never sitting still, he also was a frequent head banger, and nearly constant screamer. It didn't surprise me to hear that he had never had any coherent speech, as that is so often linked to head banging and screaming. In my opinion and experience, I believe that the head banging especially is mostly an expression of frustration. I think we can all relate to how frustrating it is when we want to express ourselves but are unable to. Who among us has not wanted to scream or vent when we can't think of that right word or name? Now imagine going through that about everything and all the time!

Despite the fact that Paul had no speech and could not write, Mom said that she knew for a fact that he "is very smart" and it was just his very poor fine motor skills that were holding him back. Great. More frustration. No wonder he's such a wiggle worm.

As with many autistic kids, one of the issues Paul's parents were most concerned about was his impulse control. Since he had almost no awareness of his surroundings and did not take direction from his parents, this can be very dangerous. Not only will children like this just run into the street, they also have no awareness of "stranger danger" and unfortunately, some strangers are a danger.

Since they had been living with the typical SAD American diet of toaster waffles and convenience foods, this was going to be quite an undertaking for them. This necessitated that Mom and I had a lengthy discussion on how and what to eat. The majority of the kids I see could probably be called picky eaters, but we had the added difficulty that Paul had a very low appetite and usually had to be coerced to eat anything at all. I encouraged her to just keep putting the right foods in front of him and just like anyone else, when he finally got hungry enough he'd eat. The proliferation of Paleo recipe websites, many of which can be used with little or no change, has made this transition immensely easier.

One-month progress report:

As is the case with lots of kids, this process did not start out easy. There were numerous bouts of crying, head banging and tantrums in response to this new way of eating. Just as his parents were questioning the wisdom of staying on the Protocol through so much drama, all of a sudden Paul began to eat. And eat. *And eat!* Going from extremely picky and with little to no appetite, they now had a chow machine on their hands. Mom described his newfound appetite as "voracious," often shoveling in three eggs, meat and vegetables for breakfast, then being the first one at the table ready for lunch.

Although this surprised them, it didn't faze me because I hear this all the time. Very young kids in particular seem to have an inherent awareness as to what is good for them; this "nature" often gets lost in the sugar addictions that most people seem to have and the kids get raised with. I have seen many children who have been raised with very little sugar in their diets who actively dislike sugar. Once they get past the "habits" of bread, sugar and other convenience foods, their bodies will actually crave the nutrient-dense food that the Protocol offers. Because of his previous diet, Paul had not been truly "fed" throughout all his four years and was clearly making up for lost time. An interesting footnote to this, is that in all the kids I have seen who went through this voracious eating phase, I've never seen one who gained any unhealthy weight. Not one. I've seen lots of kids who gained healthy weight, or more commonly went through a growth spurt, and some who dropped unhealthy weight while in this phase, but never a downside. As I said -- children do know innately what they need.

As soon as Paul started eating the "best choice" foods, the changes in him began almost immediately. Not only was he "much more comfortable in his body" he had suddenly become "cuddly and affectionate" to the joy of his family. Because of this new comfort level, he was able to sit still much longer and was sleeping better, making both him and his family a whole lot calmer and happier.

Since the families see the kids every day, and I only see them once a month, the changes are often much more apparent to me, since I've had no opportunity to "get used to them." This is why I ask people to keep a journal to better track their children's progress. While walking up to my office from the waiting room, Mom was describing initiating the diet, so I was giving my attention to her and hadn't yet taken a good look at Paul.

Even when the kids are non-verbal I talk to them and ask questions constantly, so as soon as we sat down in my office I asked him, "So how's my man Paul today?" He looked up from a toy in his hands and replied, "I like coming here, Dr. Shauna Young." A sentence. Very clear, very coherent, polite, and expressing emotion -- and knowing my formal name! Amazing.

I have to admit I was a bit shocked that Mom had not immediately mentioned Paul had begun talking, but as I said above, the family had just got used to his progress during the last month. A far cry from being non-verbal a month prior, he certainly was an exuberant little chatterbox this whole appointment!

It's been proven to me repeatedly that people definitely have different levels of enthusiasm, so I need to ask a lot of specific questions; this is one reason that I keep such detailed notes. For example, when I ask how it's going and the reply is, "Fine," I've learned that my level of fine is not necessarily a parent's level of fine. Through specific questioning I found out that in addition to his speech presenting, sentences and all, he had also suddenly potty trained himself over the course of three days with no instruction. His very poor motor skills had improved to the point that he was "tracing lines he couldn't even look at before." Wow. That's a lot of "fine" in my opinion!

As I suspected, as soon as his speech came on and he could express himself, the head banging, screaming and escaping from the house decreased, then stopped. He was listening and minding his parents much better, and when they explained why he couldn't just run out in the street, he agreed that it was a bad idea. Point: He could now be reasoned with, which was a big load about the danger issues off their minds.

Before they left, I asked Paul if he wanted to ask me anything. He thought about it for a moment then asked, "Is this good for us?" I assured him that is was very good. He took another thoughtful pause, stood up and gathered his toys and said, "Alright then. Thanks." He then gave me a very adult and serious nod, and took his leave.

Very fine indeed.

Two-month progress report:

WHOOPS!

As it so often happens, it was decided in his household that since Paul was doing so well, it would be okay to eat some foods that were off the Protocol. Despite the fact that he was progressing so rapidly, they decided it couldn't hurt to occasionally let him have some "avoid" foods. Surely, one little ol' hamburger bun won't do anything, right?

Wrong.

Soon after Paul ate that one hamburger bun his parents immediately noticed his old symptoms again rearing their ugly heads. He got very agitated and again lost his ability to focus and maintain eye contact. Fortunately, he maintained his potty training! As soon as they went back on the Protocol he rapidly reverted to his previous great gains, and had since made some additional ones. Predictably, his appetite was no longer "voracious" and was now "normal." I believe the kids just need some time to catch up on their nutrients before their appetite returns to normal.

To be honest, this kind of stuff happens a lot and I've come to believe that it's not a bad thing at all. If people are not completely convinced for some reason that the positive changes can be attributed to the Protocol, there is nothing like a slip-up and the attendant reappearance of symptoms to provide absolute proof. They were now one-hundred percent on board with the Protocol for Paul and for themselves.

All my questions about sleep, focus, fine motor skills, etc. kept yielding the same validating response: "Good, as long as he's on the Protocol." Good enough for me.

<u>Follow up:</u>

After a month steadily back on the Protocol his mom called to say that everything was back to normal and she did not feel they needed to schedule another follow-up appointment. When I talked to her almost a year later about another matter I asked how Paul was. She responded that he was "doing great." Not "fine," great. Although I'm fine with "fine," I prefer "great!"

CASE STUDY 14

Dad: *"It's nice to know we can pinpoint his behavior to food."*

Notes:

Have avoided getting any kind of DX —
He's a huge control freak —
He says, "rules are boring" and "it's easier to be bad"
He can behave if he wants something
Tells "tall tall tales" — (tells a long story about being stuck in a closet - never happened)
worries about parents getting killed
School says "non-compliance"

Name: Jamie J. (Male)

Age: 6
DX: "We're too afraid to get one"
Other diets: None. Lots of junk food.

Like many of the kids I see, the only reason there was no official diagnosis for him is because they were literally "too afraid to get one". I included Jamie as a case study for two big reasons. First: We got a very rapid and extreme reversal with his issues. Second: **Because this case clearly outlines the necessity to stay with the Protocol! If they had not changed the course they were on, thinking it would be fine to have "cheats," this would have never worked.** It is an important lesson.

Jamie had started out life very well. He walked and talked early and seemed to be on a bright track. Then shortly after a round of vaccines, his parents noticed that he started "to go off." With his infant diet of soy-based baby formulas, then having either cereal or oatmeal every morning after weaning off the formulas, it's no wonder that the manganese floodgates opened. By age three, his parents could not deny that something was definitely wrong. At first it wasn't anything they could put a finger on, he was just "different" from other children. It started with him having very involved dreams that he could describe in intricate detail. Then he began coming home from school and telling his mom that everyone was "mad at him" or that "they hated him." It was hard to figure out.

Then the lies started. At first they seemed more like imaginative "tall tales," but Jamie quickly became a skilled and pathological liar, spinning plot lines that would take thirty minutes or more to complete. When a particularly heinous one, where he told his mom that his teacher had locked him in a closet sent her running to the school, she realized how competent his lying had become. Against all logic she had believed him, primarily because of all the detail he included in his story. When she asked him why he had lied, and explained that things like that could have actually hurt the teacher's career, he laughed, flippantly commenting, "It's fun to get people in trouble."

Over time, Jamie became "a huge control freak." Things had to be completely his way at home, school, everywhere. The school said he was "non compliant" but it was more than that. The reason he didn't do as he was asked is because he simply didn't want to. It had nothing to do with focus and everything to do with control. Knowing how much his acting out in public embarrassed his parents was, by his own admission, a huge source of pleasure for him. As a result they were very limited in where they could take him. "He can behave if he wants something, so he's doing it on purpose" his mom said. Jamie arrogantly smiled at her comment.

So I asked him straight out, "If you can behave yourself if you want something, why don't you do it all the time?" His answer was right out of the control freak handbook. Very smugly and with a smirk on his face, he told me, "Rules are boring. It's easier to be bad." Yikes. Talk about a narcissist in the making! After talking with this young boy for an hour, I honestly feel that if we had not gotten this kid's issues straightened out his future might have included a jail cell. Even at this young age he had some of the very pronounced and recognizable symptoms of a sociopath.

Although his parents had heard about my Protocol months earlier from a friend, they had not considered it until recent events convinced them that they "had to do something." His control issues were continuing to escalate to the point that he was now becoming violent. He had been caught multiple times in the last few months verbally and physically bullying his brother and purposely kicking the family cat. As much as they didn't want to get him diagnosed, they were losing all their options. The Protocol felt like it was (say it with me) their last resort.

This one was going to be tough. Not only did I have a kid who enjoyed causing trouble and "being bad," and who couldn't care less about being disciplined, I had some very seriously horribly eating parents. Lots of drive through, frozen dinners, junk food and soda. When I asked what they ate when they did cook at home, his mom said "mostly quesadillas." Wow. When you think of melting packaged individually wrapped cheese slices onto a store-bought tortilla in a microwave as "home cooking" we've got some serious trouble.

Both parents were significantly overweight and unhealthy, and were visibly freaked out by the idea that they would have to actually cook real food in the house. Dad, who had been pretty onboard up until this point, went off the rails when I told him that the whole family needed to be on the Protocol together. Being a hardcore sugar and junk food junkie, he got very defensive at this point. Finally he said to his wife, "If you and Jamie want to do it you can. I'm not." I explained to him how and why it would desperately compromise the chances of the Protocol succeeding if he still had junk food in the house that Jamie could get to. Again he shook me off. Waving a hand at his wife he said "That's your problem then."

In watching his reactions, it quickly became obvious that Jamie was actively enjoying the conflict, not only between his parents, but especially between me and his dad. He was following the conversation closely and every time I would get close to us agreeing on something, Jamie would interject a comment to fan the flames again. Just as his dad was getting to the point of agreeing to at least try it, Jamie would say something like "Are you going let her tell you what to do? Who is she to do that?" and away we'd go again. Each time he did this he would turn to me with a very self-satisfied "take that" smile and faux-innocent expression. Though not exactly a technical term, it was actually creepy how skilled he was at creating and controlling conflict, and how much he loved rubbing it in my face that he could. And coming from a six-year-old? Yuck.

Knowing a sugar addict when I see one, I now concentrated my efforts on Mom instead of Dad. In addition to Jamie's issues, she had been struggling with weight and some other health problems herself for many years. I encouraged her to join Jamie on the Protocol not only for him, but for her sake, and explained the many benefits of a Paleo diet; as the Protocol is a targeted, but Paleo, diet. I guided her to some of my favorite Paleo recipe websites, and gave her some recipes that people on the Protocol had created and shared with me over the years. By the time they left I hoped that I had talked her off the ledge, but you never know. Dad was already in the car so I didn't expect much help there.

1.5-month progress report:

There had been a lot of ups and downs this month, but just at my first glance I saw some ups. I know it may make me sound a bit wimpy, especially when you're talking about a six-year-old boy, but Jamie's intensity the month before had been chilling. It was too much like one of those horror movies with kids talking in rhymes or something. Today, when I went to greet them in the waiting room, Jaime smiled and asked me how my day was going. This appointment took place in November so he asked me polite questions about what my favorite season was, and admired the view of the snow dusting on the mountains from my second-story office before taking his seat.

The Protocol, as I had predicted, had been a huge change for them and Mom was really struggling to figure out what to cook. Her husband remained firmly *not* on board, and that definitely complicated the mix for both her and Jamie. She had remained determined though and they had made some excellent headway. Jamie was *doing* better, and she was *feeling* better.

As so often happens, especially with the more ODD (Oppositional Defiance Disorder) and violent natured kids, he actually got a little worse the first week or so into the Protocol, then abruptly did a 180 and started making positive change. His behavior in general had become "so much better" and thankfully the attacks on his brother and the cat had stopped. "We went three weeks with no problems at all. It was amazing," his mother noted.

So here comes the hammer. Because Jamie was doing so well, they figured that it was okay to not only let him go trick or treating, but to eat his entire haul of candy Halloween night. What was one splurge, right? Oh, so wrong! "One night of all that candy and we had our nightmare back," Mom admitted. It's amazing how much of not only sugar but wheat there is in candy! Wheat!

After going strictly back to Phase 1 of the Protocol for a week, Jamie started to settle back down. He went right back to being much calmer and compliant, and once again the elaborate lies ceased. You would think that this experience would have been enough to convince his parents that it was the food behind Jamie's devilish behavior, but apparently not. Shortly after getting him straightened out again, Jamie came down with a cold and told his mom that the only food he was willing to eat was quesadillas. He stuck to his guns, she caved in, and quesadillas it was for two days.

Predictably, their "nightmare" as his mother described it, came roaring back. Again. And as soon as they went back on Phase 1, the good behavior returned. Again.

This example shows the absolute power of food addictions -- and just how intensely diet affects behavior. Although they could see for themselves that Jamie did incredibly well on the Protocol, and became violent and controlling off the Protocol, they still allowed him his "splurges." Why would they do that? My opinion is that it has more to do with themselves than their child. The idea that their own indulgences that are "once in a while" or "just a little" are okay, get blown out of the water in the face of this kind of hard and fast evidence. This is particularly tough to take when you have heavily defended food addictions of your own.

Being that "the holidays" were just around the corner, I told them that they would have to be extra vigilant with Jamie's diet. It's funny. I always enjoyed this time of year until I started this line of work. While it's fun to be in the holiday spirit and visit friends and family, that time of year can be a land mine when it comes to staying on your diet, and I often spend January and February helping people mop up their various damage. Jamie's parents assured me that would not be the case. Truthfully, I had my doubts.

Two-month progress report:

They had been as good as their word, and Jamie's behavior was reflecting their added diligence. He was doing "really really really good" proclaimed his exuberant mom, and he was making new progress. The bullying and the lies that had been so concerning were gone, and he had decided that he wanted to start playing on the basketball team at school.

The control issues had also lessened considerably. "He still has some on occasion," his mom reported, "but he's a lot less argumentative." Obviously, he still had some work to do in that area, but I am open to the idea that some people just want more control over their situations than others. It's my belief that it is more a matter of inherent personality than health. As long as it wasn't resulting in heated arguments or physical violence, I had confidence that it was something they could manage.

When I asked if there was anything left to work on, his mom said she felt that any issues left were "nothing that isn't regular six-year-old stuff." Feeling that they learned from his food-related melt-downs, and now being safely past the holidays, I felt that they could handle the rest on their own, and thus discharged him on Phase 3 of the Protocol. Wrong again.

Three months later: (phone)

In came the panicked phone call. Because he was doing so well, Jamie's parents again decided that they "didn't need to be so strict." Jamie had asked if he could have toast with peanut butter for breakfast so they agreed to let him have "a little."

Knowing the treat he wanted was in the house, Jamie went into the kitchen early the next morning and ate half a loaf of white bread with peanut butter in one sitting. So much for "a little". If it had indeed been "a little" he probably wouldn't have such an extreme reaction. But since it was "a lot" and more particularly, a lot of bread, he blew up. By the time the rest of the family got out of bed he was already into a full on melt-down.

In the following days he went right back to his old tricks of arguing, lying and bullying. As if this weren't enough, in addition to the old symptoms he also got several new ones; including a red, itchy rash extending from below his nostrils to his chin, uncontrolled head twitching, and he started wetting the bed. At this point, even Jamie had to admit that his food cravings were the basis of his issues. As his mom said, "At least now he admits he's had bad food instead of lying."

Her next question of "What do we do now?" was easily answered. "You know the answer to that," I told her. She did, and they went back on Phase 1. After a single month on it, Jamie went right back to being himself (his good self, that is). "He's back doing really good," she told me on the phone. "It's actually amazing."

Silver lining:

Although this was the end of my formal dealings with Jamie, I was far from done with this family. His dad, who had commonly eaten microwave popcorn and soda as his "dinner," and rarely ate anything but fast food for lunch, came around in a big way. He became a client of mine himself and was able to lose not only weight, but successfully addressed his high blood pressure and cholesterol issues through the Paleo way of eating. According to his wife, he is still making everyone crazy at work talking about his new way of eating, and how great he feels. You probably know the joke; how can you tell if someone is eating Paleo? Don't worry, they'll tell you. He became a great example of that.

Mom, although she is still fighting the battle of carb and sugar addictions, has managed to lose over 50 pounds and is committed to the grain-free lifestyle. When she falls off the wagon, she admits it instead of making excuses, and then climbs back on. That's a huge step just in itself, and the mindset that practically guarantees long-term success. Giddy up…

Follow up:

Although I have not seen Jamie as a client since 2012, I have seen him quite a bit when he comes in with his mom or dad. The whole family is eating the Paleo way these days, including his little brother, which is probably one big reason I've never needed to see him as a client. Jamie is almost ten now, and it's hard to believe how sweet and silly he can be. He still has an amazing command of language for someone his age, but instead of using it to bully and intimidate people, he's using it to make them laugh. He is a bit of a "know it all," but don't we all know people like that? And to his credit, he does know a lot. He's really an incredibly smart kid.

CASE STUDY 15

What type? _____

Flapping and/or "stimming"?   0 1 2 3 4 5 6 7 8 9 10

Hits themselves and/or head banging?   Hyperactive, need constant attention at times

What else do we need to know about your child? Gets extremely angry.
Kicks, bangs, screams when he doesn't get
Something he wants, doesn't like being alone, rocks
a lot of attention, wheat/sugar make him
act crazy/disobedient/hyperactive. He's doing well too
in school though. If there has been too
much activity, or wrong foods he is restless and
night and can't get to sleep, his whole body seems
to be twitching, uncomfortable.

Rev 080924

Name: Sean T. (Male)
Age: 5
DX: Sensory Integration Disorder
Other diets: None

It never ceases to amaze me how *different* all the kids I see are from
each other. The idea of "acting like a five-year-old" is a farfetched
idea at best for the most part, but when you throw in the effects of
Menefe Syndrome then you have a whole different can of worms.
This guy was like no five-year-old I've ever seen.

As so many of the kids I've worked with are, there was no question
that Sean was vastly intelligent. He had the vocabulary of an adult,
but spoke in an odd slurred fashion, and would utter inappropriate or
irrelevant sentences for no particular reason. And he never stopped

talking! The entire hour of our first appointment was punctuated by his never-ceasing ramblings and nonsensical chatter. I don't know when he took time to breathe!

When his mother was talking to me about her and her husband's biggest concern, which was his "instant anger," Sean abruptly chimed in, "It's a weird thing with me; if I don't get everything I want then I get very mad and throw a fit. My body just tells me to." When I asked him if he felt that was the correct response, he snapped, "I don't care if it is or not."

According to Mom's description, her son could be set off by just about anything (or nothing) and could become quite violent in his tantrums. During the appointment when she was describing an incident that had occurred because the pair of jeans Sean wanted to wear that day were currently in the laundry basket, he jumped up and yelled at her, "I won't wear anything that isn't hip and cool!" This behavior, which I would consider to be inappropriate in a teenager, was even more baffling to see in a five-year-old. Hip and cool? I expected his mom to address the fact that he had just gotten up in her face and screamed at her, but she just said "I know, buddy." Buddy? Uh oh.

Warning. Some of you may get a tad angry at me at this point, but that's just a chance I'm going to have to take. As much as I don't wish to criticize anyone's parenting techniques, and fully respect the rights of parents to decide what is good and not good for their kids, this "buddy" or "pal" or "chum" thing is a real buzzkill for me. Fact: I've seen this one thing ruin the kids' recovering more times than I can count. It came into play so much in this case that it still shocks me to this day that we had the outstanding outcome we did. Here's why it rankles: When you call your child a term that is synonymous with "friend," the child believes he or she is indeed more a "friend" than a child. As such, the power base shifts more toward the child and his/her demands. In these cases it usually follows that the necessary instructive discipline also tends to be erratic, non-existent, or lackluster in delivery. Not a hip or cool family dynamic in my book. Kids can have other kids as friends. They need parents to be parents.

Sean's mom believed that the best course of action for him was to be able to "express himself" and enforced little to no discipline over him (no longer a surprise). During the course of the appointment, he frequently yelled at her, called her "stupid," and was generally completely disrespectful to her. If she wanted to deal with that, it was her business and not mine, but when he tried it with me, proclaiming me to be "just another idiot" I put a stop to it. I reprimanded, "Sean, you will not speak to me like that. It's disrespectful and I won't have it."

As shocked as he was, it didn't even compare to his mother's reaction. She was very upset with me because I spoke to her little "buddy" that way, and asked me to immediately apologize to him. Ignoring that, I told her that whatever he was like at home was her business, but when he was in my office he would show respect or they could take their leave. While they were still sitting there with their mouths open at my audacity, I turned and looked little Sean right in the eye. I asked, "Are we clear on this?" He gulped a few times and sheepishly stammered, "Yes, Ma'am" and that was the end of that. I can't imagine what working with him would have been like without that meeting of the minds.

We had a lot to address here. In addition to his violent anger, he was also hugely hyperactive and was constantly drumming his hands on everything, tapping his feet, and would have episodes of head banging that his parents had a hard time stopping. Add this to the incessant talking, talking, talking and he was like a one-man band. This hyperactivity spilled over into his bedtimes and he had a particularly hard time getting to sleep. To further complicate this, he refused to even try to sleep at all unless his mother was physically in the room with him all night.

As much as the manganese imbalance, I believe much of this hyperactivity was closely linked to his severe sugar addiction. Yes, addiction. Even for a child, Sean had one of the most severe sugar addictions I've ever seen, and his behavior would quickly escalate when he would be denied it. After five pieces of licorice that his mother had given him thus far in the appointment, he was demanding a sixth. When she timidly said she thought he'd had enough for now, he leaped up screaming obscenities at her and began banging his hands and head against the floor to ceiling glass windows of my second-story office. As soon as she acquiesced and quickly brought out another piece of candy, he stopped yelling and sat back down, quiet as could be. That reaction my friends, is a sure sign of addiction. He had ten pieces of licorice during the one-hour appointment. In addition to everything else, this sugar addiction of his and his mom's acquiescence to it did not bode well for hopes of following the Protocol!

In addition to his fears of the dark and of being alone, Sean was also afraid of many ordinary things. Little things like animals, neighbors, or sounds when he couldn't immediately identify the source. He could not stand anything noisy whatsoever and would "spin out of control" not only at home, but virtually anywhere, like in the car or at the grocery store. He was teased at school because his virtually nonexistent fine motor skills did not allow him to be able to catch a ball, or even use a knife and fork.

When we began going over the specific foods of the Protocol the tempest really began. Sean immediately began yelling at the top of his lungs, "Noooo! I don't like this! This is terrifying me! Noooo!" while his tearful mom (seriously, she was crying) apologized over and over to her "buddy" for "making him eat this terrible diet." When I asked what part she thought was "terrible" about it, it was as I suspected -- it was food instead of sugar. Mom voiced her concern that he would "starve to death" since he currently ate very little of what was on the Protocol-allowed foods. I assured her that as long as the good foods were all that was in the house, he would get hungry and eat it. He of course, seconded the motion that he "would starve and die" on this. They were both crying and seemed to be approaching some hysterics at this point, so I left the room for a moment to allow them to calm down.

When I came back in, I calmly told his mother that this is what I had to offer them. A diet. If they didn't want to try it, then that was completely up to them. I did make it clear that I wasn't interested in any more tantrums from either of them. Mom agreed that "she and Sean would discuss it" so I figured that this would be the last I would ever see of them. He wanted no part of it, and I couldn't see her pushing it.

Once again, I was wrong. Only this time, I was happy to be wrong.

One-month progress report:

Since Sean's father is a hunter and they had a large supply of local bison and elk in their home, he thought that it would be a great idea to at least try the Protocol, since they had such high-quality proteins easily at hand. I would never meet Dad, or even learn his name, but his son has a lot to thank him for.

To his mother's complete surprise, things were "much better." Sean's white-hot anger had cooled to "flashes" of temper that were not nearly as intense or as frequent as before. After the initial tantrums (and withdrawal symptoms) about receiving so much less sugar, he calmed down almost immediately. The tantrums returned briefly, and his mom found that they were related to the fact that he had been sneaking into the kitchen at night and drinking almost a gallon of apple juice. Sugar is a horrible addiction, and Sean had some hard detoxing to do, but at least things were calming down.

When I asked Sean for his feelings about how things were going, he too felt that his situation was improving. In his odd, slurred speech he admitted, "I'm a lot calmer. I used to shout 'I'm lonely' at bed-time every night. I don't do that anymore." His sleep in general was more restful, and he was sleeping alone in his room with just a small nightlight. As it turns out, Mom sleeping in his room every night had caused some friction in her marriage, so everyone was feeling happi-er.

When I asked if there was any improvement in his fine motor skills, Mom replied she "didn't know." I reminded her that it was most easily gauged by how well he was using utensils, and she explained, "He likes eating with his hands and I'm just letting him do what feels right to him." Putting aside the social aspects of a five-year-old eating with his hands at a gathering or restaurant (again, not my busi-ness), I told her that it would be hard to assess any progress he was able to make if she wasn't monitoring it. She and Sean discussed it and agreed that they would try it for that reason.

At the end of the appointment she asked Sean if he wanted to stay on the Protocol for another month. He said, "Let's see how I feel about it," and she agreed. I wasn't hazarding any guesses this time.

Two-month progress report:

In starting back to school, the Protocol apparently had not felt good to Sean because with his pretzel, cracker, candy and cookie eating, we were all the way back to square one. When I asked his mom why she had allowed all the progress he had made to be lost, simply for the sake of snacks, she told me, "I'm afraid of making him feel controlled and stigmatized. He's making his own choice to eat them." Okay. Enough is enough. He's five!

At this point I asked Sean if he would please go downstairs and get a file for me from my receptionist. My entire staff knows that this is the signal that they need to keep the kid in the waiting area if they can, because Mom and I were about to have "The Talk."

As I've stated emphatically, I actively hate getting involved in family business. How you want to raise your kids is up to you. However, when a child makes such dramatic progress I feel that it is my duty as their doctor to advocate for that child to the best of my abilities. I had my usual "You're his mother not his buddy" talk, but while we were having this conversation I noticed a strange attitude from her. It became quickly apparent that she was, in small ways but there nonetheless, sabotaging him. I asked her, "Do you feel that you may have any attachment to the idea of him not growing up and becoming more like other kids?" The answer was telling: "You sound just like my husband. That's what he always says." Hmmm. Score another point for Dad.

Three-month progress report:

Deciding to be "sticklers" on the Protocol this month had done a world of good. Sean not only regained all the ground he had lost the previous month, he had made some new progress. He was still chatty, but the constant endless dialogue was gone, and when he did speak it was pertinent to what was being discussed. Although he said he was tired of the diet because "It's all meat and vegetables" he did acknowledge that he felt it was doing him a lot of good.

As I mentioned, the first time I saw Sean I noticed that he had a very strange slurring sound to his voice. Up to this point, this had never changed and I was thinking about recommending that his parents get his hearing checked as he sounded very much like a friend of mine who is deaf. She jokes that she went to one of the most expensive schools in the world so that she could "wind up sounding like a drunk," and is that is how Sean sounded. This appointment however, I noticed that the odd slurring was much less noticeable.

The parents had decided to test his fine motor skills out, and Sean had found it a surprisingly easy matter to start using a knife and fork. Nearly at the same time his balance had unexpectedly improved and he was riding a bicycle and getting into some sports at school. It's amazing how often the motor skills and balance seem to go hand-in-hand and to come together at the same time.

He was sleeping well, and by himself, and was feeling calmer without the fears and loneliness that always plagued him especially at bedtime. He was becoming much more involved at school, making new friends, and his grades were improving.

When I asked about the anger and tantrums, his mother perked up. "It's so much better. Yesterday he got zapped by a false friend and there was a ton of bad energy but he got through it fine. I'm going to take him to a class about energies anyway." Yes, that's really a quote. You can't make this stuff up. To this comment Sean rolled his eyes and replied "That sounds fun." Okay, he was being sarcastic, but at least he smiled when he said it and wasn't disrespectful or mean about it.

Even though he was doing so well, I still suggested they come back one more time to make sure that the new changes would stick with him this time. Mom predictably said it was up to him, and Sean felt that was reasonable.

Four-month progress report:

With another month gone, Sean was still doing great. The rages and tantrums were gone and with it the kinetic hyperactivity that had fueled his constant movements and chatter. He felt calm, was sleeping well, and his irrational fears had dissolved. Far from his original trepidations, he was becoming a bit adventurous and was making some preliminary attempts to spread his wings. He loved riding his bike, and was now wanting to ride it back and forth to his neighborhood school alone.

His speech, which had improved the month before, had now lost all of the strangeness I had originally noticed. He was speaking faster, and his words sounded crisp and normal. When I remarked on this improvement, Mom said, "I don't notice those kinds of things. I just love him the way he is." Sean once again rolled his eyes but held his peace. He had definitely acquired some self-control.

When I asked if they felt there was anything left to work on, they both said that they felt everything was "great." I like great! I told them that although Sean would still need to stay away from sugars and grains, they would no longer need to be on the Protocol as strictly, and could progress to a more Paleo-style diet. With this news, Sean jumped out of his chair and exclaimed "Wait... I can still have salmon and mangos can't I"? This from a five-year-old who formerly ate little but sugar. Mom assured the once-picky eater, that yes, salmon and mangos could still be on the menu.

Follow-up:

I discharged Sean from our monthly visits in May 2009. As I had expected, he turned out to be not only unusually intelligent, but very creative. As time went on, his intellect continued to show itself and I would, without hesitation, call him a genius.

There is a humorous (to me at least) end note to this story. Several years down the road, I got a panicked phone call from Sean's mom telling me that he had "regressed and was becoming autistic again" and that they needed to get in immediately. This seemed odd for many reasons, including the fact that his diagnosis had been Sensory Integration Disorder and not autism, and because it is highly unusual for someone to regress. When I asked for details about this regression, she informed me that he and a few other boys had written a rather mild four-letter word on a wall at school. You know, the S word. Trying hard not to laugh I gave her my take on the situation. "Sorry, Mom. That's not autism. That's being eight."

CHAPTER SEVEN

Autistic Behavior vs. Kid Behavior

It has long been said that the only thing that is constant is change. It is normal also for many people to resist it, especially if they do not expect circumstances to transform their lives so significantly. The key here is learning what to anticipate and to cultivate an understanding that change will happen, so you can adapt more easily to it.

As your child on the Protocol begins to respond physically, mentally and emotionally as symptoms subside, it is vital that you respond and change with him or her. Many of the kids have such rapid progress that it can put you and other family members into a real tailspin, so you have to be ready to keep up! We tend to build our own behaviors from what we have come to expect from the pre-Protocol child and thus become used to our own behaviors as "normal" responses.

Now you have to go to work on your own mindset as a parent and learn to differentiate between "autistic behavior" and "kid behavior." This is especially true with the older children, as they have developed lifelong patterns in how they go about their lives and they are just as reluctant to change them as we adults are. If a tantrum in the grocery store has always produced the desired results of a candy bar, chances are they will continue to use this behavior, as it's always been successful. Just realize that what you have is no longer an uncontrollable autistic child, and you will probably need to develop some different tools of parental discipline to change your new child's previous bad habits. Parents often wind up changing just as much as their kids with this Protocol!

Previously non-verbal children who have learned to sign often have to be reminded to "use their words" instead of signing or pointing. The older they are and the longer they have been using sign language the more likely it is that they will fall back on it. This is especially important if you have other children in the family since many times the other siblings have grown used to being facilitators for the "special needs" child, and are always "interpreting" for them.

Very often I suggest that parents start assigning their children "ownership" tasks at this point; such as setting the table, taking out the garbage, or helping fold laundry. Many of these kids have never had to ask for anything because the family, out of love, has tried to anticipate their needs and will not initiate doing more without being prompted. I remember a particular case where the mom said she knew her autistic son was getting better in an amusing way. He was whining from his bedroom to his older sister, who was in her bedroom, that he wanted something from the kitchen and she yelled, "Go get it yourself!" And he did. As I said, progress doesn't always look the way you think it will.

Having said this, it is also important to remember that your child does and should have their own personality and it might not be exactly what you were anticipating. For example, if your child is not where you think they should be with social interaction, this may not signify autistic behavior; the kid just might just naturally be shy and reserved! Instead of assuming that it is a symptom of some kind, try asking your child *why* he or she avoids certain situations or people.

On the other side of the spectrum, several years after a boy I worked with graduated from the Protocol, I received a panicked phone call from his mother who said her son was "going autistic" again. Why? Because he and a few friends had chalked a four-letter word on a wall at school. Sorry Mom. That's not autistic, that's just being eight!

Another time I had a case where the parents were concerned that their ten and twelve year old boys, who were doing fantastic, were "still autistic" because they were not getting straight A's! Again, sorry Mom. There isn't a diet in the world that will do that! Boys will be boys and they were much more interested in getting dirty by running around and playing than in getting straight A's.

One of my pet peeves is when autistic children are clumped together and referred to generically as "these kids." As in "These kids are all low in iron," or "These kids" all think or behave the same way. They are not "these kids!" They are Joe and Sarah and Logan and Lily and they are as different in personality as snowflakes. Don't fall into that trap yourself! They're your kids.

Many people seem to think that they need to be giving their children a lot supplements, and although I do often use a very few targeted supplements, please remember *that this is all about the food.* Supplements can have some benefit in some cases, but there are often downsides. As an example, I had a mother who was very nervous about taking her four-year-old off the seventeen supplements she was currently on because her daughter was "much calmer" while taking them. So I asked her to try an experiment for me. Although she out-weighed her daughter by nearly one hundred pounds, I asked her to take the exact same dosage of supplements suggested for her daughter herself for two days and then call me back. When she called and I asked her how she felt, she predictably said "nauseous." Her daughter wasn't calmer - she was nauseous! Is that how you want your kids to feel? Of course not. But since her child was non-verbal at the time she couldn't tell Mom she just didn't feel good.

The only hard and fast rule of the Spectrum Balance Protocol is that it has to be strictly adhered to until the imbalance is cor-

rected. I have seen months of progress be heartbreakingly ruined by the most seemingly small things. One bowl of cereal. One cupcake. One weekend at Grandma's, who insists that "a few cookies can't possibly hurt anything." I know it sounds crazy, and I know I repeat this, but I've seen it happen over and over. Get in it for the long haul and just think -- maybe if you skip Halloween candy or a birthday cake this year, you won't have to worry about it by next year. Isn't that worth some extra effort?

16 - 20

One of the (many) circumstances that we never anticipated encountering was regarding the parents reaction to their children changing so dramatically and so quickly. The kids themselves rarely have any problem with it and just take it in stride, especially the little ones. But if you're a parent it can cause some emotional whiplash.

Many of these families have spent numerous years - often the span of the child's entire life - worrying, obsessing and hovering over their every move. So when your child suddenly matures, sometimes many years at a jump, and starts wanting their own space, it's hard to know how to react. However, if your family is on this Protocol, you may need to get ready to fasten your seat-belts.

Here are a few of the kids who made these huge leaps, including one amazing guy who continues to insist to his school, his family, and pretty much everyone, that he is "not special". I happen to think he's very special; but not because of autism.

CASE STUDY 16

Mom: *"He is so, so, so good now! I can't thank you enough!"*

Name: Ryan G. (Male)

Age: 13
DX: Autism
RX: Armour and Zoloft. At least twelve nutritional supplements recommended by a variety of specialists
Other diets: GFCF, GAPS, Vegan, SCD
ND: Linda Kane

At the age of three, a developmental pediatrician had diagnosed Ryan as "severely autistic and severely retarded" and advised that his parents consider putting him in a group home for the rest of his life as he would "never function independently." Quite a statement regarding a three-year-old. Unwilling to accept this sentence, his family began working with a series of behavioral specialists, and started doing a trial program in which Ryan received forty hours a week of ABA therapy, speech therapy, and occupational therapy.

Under this guidance, he made enough significant improvement to be able to start at a private pre-school with the help of an aide. By the next year he was doing well enough that he went on to kindergarten and then first grade, always continuing with his aide. Already he was proving his original diagnosis as… well… extreme.

All went fairly well until he was six-and-a-half when he got a series of routine vaccinations. Immediately afterward, the sweet and loving boy became an altogether different person. It started out with him having a what appeared to be a psychotic break -- pretending to be someone else, making up imaginary people and acting out badly enough that the school called to find out what had happened. This odd behavior progressed quickly and he became very aggressive and sometimes even violent. He pulled people's hair at school, and began pinching, kicking and hitting his family members. As his mom put it: "It was so frightening, because we didn't know how to help him or what was the cause."

Their desperation to find solutions led his parents to try many therapies, including Hyperbaric Oxygen Therapy (HBOT) to increase the flow of oxygen to his brain. After the first few dives (as an HBOT treatment is called), they saw enough improvement to continue. He did two dives a week for a total of 116 treatments.

Eventually between the HBOT, chelation therapy designed to remove any heavy metals from his system, and Bioresonance treatments, Ryan finally began to settle down, returning to his former gentle self.

Even though he was ranked behaviorally at a four to five-year-old level, his mind was far beyond that. At the age of only ten, he hacked into a business school website and filled out an application to their school of computer science and technology! His mother didn't know about this until she got a call from the program director. More intrigued than angry, the director wanted to talk to Ryan about his "creative" application that had apparently used some very sophisticated patterning techniques. Imagine the director's shock when he found out that Ryan was autistic… and ten!

Since the HBOT treatments had brought about such positive advancements, Ryan's parents decided to do another round of them. On the first day, his mom went into the hyperbaric chamber with him as she usually did. Normally, when you do HBOT therapy the pressure in the chamber is released very slowly at the end of the treatment to allow the people inside to equalize the pressure their body has been under. This time, for some reason, the pressure was taken off very quickly and Mom noticed she had an immediate nasty headache. She addressed this quick exit with the technician and asked for the pressure to be taken off much more slowly on the second dive. Because of her headache, Dad went in with Ryan for his second dive. For some reason, the HBOT technician did not heed the request and again, took the pressure off very quickly.

After that day, Ryan was not the same again. That very night, his entire body lit up with pain and he could not stop urinating. The doctor whose HBOT tank they used adamantly denied that the two events were connected, and Ryan's parents were once again struggling to find out how to help him.

Trips to his pediatrician (who said it was "all in his head") and a pediatric urologist yielded no answers. Although Ryan continued in constant aching pain and was making in excess of twenty trips to the bathroom, just during school hours alone, all the doctors they saw said that they couldn't find anything physically wrong with him.

Going to yet another specialist (in California this time), he was diagnosed with "a complex autoimmune disease" and "a complex viral disease," so the doctor put him on high doses of anti-viral medications. On this treatment, Ryan became extremely weak and in such enormous pain that he missed most of the school year, and he was still urinating constantly. After six months of this regimen with no positive result, his mom started doing internet research and discovered that her already frail son was on five times the normal adult dosage of the anti-virals! Afraid of the listed side effects of liver and kidney damage, she called the doctor to air her concerns. He was very upset with her that she would "question him" and actually yelled at her before hanging up on her. Mom said, "It was at this point I realized that this doctor did not know what he was doing."

All the medical doctors they saw all said the same thing; that there was nothing physically wrong with Ryan, but obviously there was since he was in constant pain. Out of options in the standard medical world, his parents began seeking alternate therapies.

Fortunately for Ryan, his parents took him to Texas this time to see Dr. Jerry Tennant; an MD who works with integrative medicine, including Tesla and frequency light treatments. Although the boy's autism had taken a backseat to his perplexing physical issues, it was that part of his profile that caused Dr. Tennant to suggest that Ryan be put on my Protocol. Dr. Tennant was very familiar with my work, as he had taken the time to come out to Colorado and learn about it in the prior year and has advised it to many of his patients. After doing a series of pain treatments with him, they headed back home and immediately started the Protocol.

Within ten days, Ryan's situation was already changing. The constant debilitating pain that he had constantly been in for over two years was quickly receding, and the frequent urination was steadily lessening. At long last, something was working! This was enough ammunition for them to get on a plane once more to fly all the way across the country to see yet another specialist. This time the specialist was me.

By the time I actually saw Ryan, he was no longer in pain. In the few short weeks since he had seen Dr. Tennant and had started on the Protocol they had noticed several changes. Of course, the fact that his pain disappeared was tantamount, but they also noticed other less dramatic things. He seemed calmer, he was speaking in more complete sentences, and was much easier to get along with. "We're very happy with what we're seeing so far."

When his parents told me that he was thirteen I was very surprised. Judging from his size I thought he was probably only nine or ten at most. Apparently his lifetime history of illness, treatments and medications had taken a toll on the poor guy. When I met him he weighed only eighty-three pounds and had no muscle tone.

Despite being extremely intelligent, Ryan was still diagnosed behaviorally at a four to five-year-old level. Non-aware and hyperactive, he was uttering bursts of unconnected and childlike speech. His "complete lack of impulse control" showed itself when he asked my receptionist, in front of a roomful of people, if he could "squeeze her boobs." She gracefully declined. Well, at least he asked.

Since his puzzling and painful health issues had already almost completely resolved in his few weeks since Dr. Tennant's treatments and on the Protocol, Mom and Dad were very gung-ho to continue it to attempt to address his autism. We discussed the most proactive way to fit the foods he liked into the Protocol yet still achieve the best results possible. Their main issue was fruit, as Ryan wanted to eat way too much of it. It is sometimes hard to get people to understand that although fruit contains more natural sugars, it is still sugar! We set up a phone appointment for thirty days since they live on the East Coast.

One-month progress report: (phone)

Even though Ryan was dealing with a bout of pneumonia, he was still making noticeable progress. People often use that their child is sick as an excuse to not be on the Protocol, but in this case the parents stuck to their guns. When I complimented her on doing so, his mom said "Even though he's not feeling well he's doing so much better." The best news was that despite the fact that he was sick the aching had not returned, thank goodness.

With the help of his medical doctor, his parents had weaned Ryan off his prescription medications and they were very pleased with the results. As soon as they took him off the Armour they noticed that he was immediately calmer. They had been worried that they may see behavioral issues coming off the Zoloft, but in fact had noticed nothing at all either good or bad. As for the over a dozen of supplements they had been giving him, he was now down to five. This was causing his mom some anxiety that he would lose ground, but Ryan was very happy about it. Like most people he did not enjoy taking so many pills every day. He had griped about the Protocol at first, but with the payoff of taking so many fewer pills was making the meal plan easier to swallow.

Even with the relatively short time that Ryan had been on the Protocol, the changes were very noticeable. He was rapidly emerging from the haze of "non-awareness" that plagues autistic children and was entering the real world. In this month alone he had started to enjoy watching the nightly news and was asking pertinent questions about it afterward. He had begun noticing things around the house that he previously had been oblivious to, and then taking it upon himself to remedy. "He started doing chores and no one even asked him to!" said his merrily bewildered mother. I'll bet a lot of people wish their teenager would do that!

He was rapidly progressing from childlike and disconnected speech to being able to express himself much more clearly and in much richer detail. This was also helping with his impulsivity and temper because he could now say what he wanted to say instead of feeling powerless to express himself. An example of this was that a few nights before our conversation, Ryan's sister was annoying him and he calmly requested, "Will you please stop doing that" instead of reacting with his usual yelling.

While still impulsive, Mom noticed that even when he acted out in some fashion, it seemed that he was aware of it now. I told her that this would probably turn out to be the hardest part to work on, since he was thirteen and used to getting things his way. Old habits are hard to break, and he had a lot of old habits!

Two-month progress report: (phone)

During the course of this month they had been traveling quite a bit and were not as exacting on the Protocol as they had been at first. And as usual, it showed. Ryan's progress slowed, and in a few areas they'd seen some slight regression. He was more angry and tired, and his speech, which had been making huge advances, had relapsed again.

Mom made no excuses and took full responsibility for the lapses. It is harder to stay on this or any dietary Protocol when you're not at home, but it isn't impossible. You just have to plan around it more, and you may have to step on a few toes when staying with others. It always surprises me when people tell me that their relatives actually get offended if you don't eat the same way they do, but I've heard it quite often. When asked if this relapse had convinced her, her unhesitating answer was "Yes, it's more trouble. So now I don't care. No matter what happens he is staying on this diet."

Luckily something that did not relapse was his pain. He was thankfully still pain free. "I have to tell you that this is totally amazing. We've tried everything and for the first time in more than two years he's not in pain. I don't feel helpless anymore."

Three-month progress report: (phone)

A more rigorous adherence to the Protocol had brought about some major changes this month. He was doing so well both academically and more importantly, socially, at school that he was now attending school without the help of his aide for the first time in his life.

Blooming under this new feeling of independence, Ryan was now wanting to do more and more things by himself. Instead of sitting with his aide at lunch, he was now joining in at the communal lunch tables and was having full and complete conversations with the other kids. While needing some time to catch up on his social skills, mostly "appropriateness," the kids were accepting him without much comment.

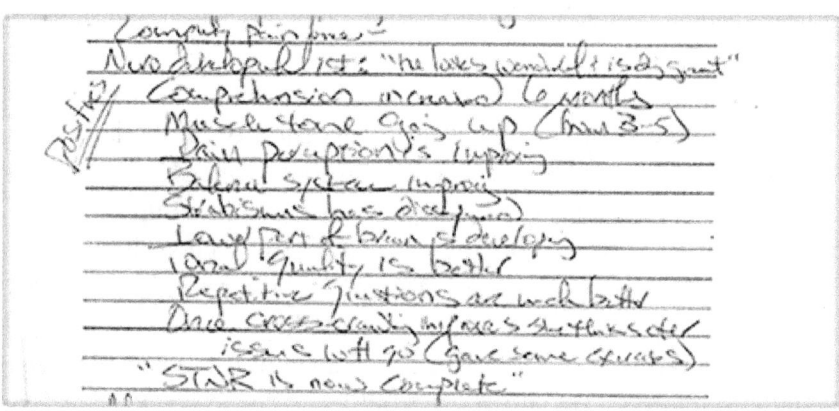

His body was feeling the effects of the Protocol as well, as he grew several inches and gained over fifteen pounds of healthy weight in what seemed like "overnight." I've seen this often where the kids go through one of these sudden growth spurts and it is usually around this same time in the third to fourth months on the Protocol. With his larger size and sudden better coordination, he had started to ice skate and was getting interested in playing ice hockey.

While Ryan was taking all these changes in stride, it was harder on his mom! Even though all the changes were positive it was a lot to absorb in such a short period of time. Her son, who had basically been hovering on the edge of death for his entire life, now wanted to walk to school alone, make his own decisions, and start living his own life. It sounds wonderful to say that behaviorally your son went from four to almost fourteen in less than four months, but imagine if that happened to you! It was now Mom's old habits that we needed to work on. We discussed the "helicopter mom" scenario, where she is constantly hovering over him, and she agreed that it certainly applied to her.

This situation, where a child I'm working with matures so suddenly that the family has difficulty adjusting, became so common that I began working with a psychologist who would do phone consultations to provide advice about how to adapt. Melaney Sreenan's skilled counseling to break old habits, with both the recovering child and the family members, has carried many families over this particular speed bump. Ryan's mother gratefully took her number.

Four-month progress report: (phone)

"He looks good and he feels good."

Those few words pretty much summed up our conversation. Ryan had gone through yet another growth spurt and was now taller than his mother and up more than twenty healthy pounds. The exercise he was getting skating was showing as he had also put on quite a bit of noticeable muscle, which he was happy to display.

School was also going very well for Ryan. His improved reading and math skills had put him on the Honor Roll, and he was becoming much more social. His social skills and "appropriateness" still needed some work but he was catching up. Getting punched by a guy at school for a social gaff probably helped this along! His ever protective mom was concerned, but Ryan himself brushed it off and bragged to me that the bruised eye made him look "manly." Getting in little scuffles like this felt like freedom to him and more than likely went a long way in showing him what was appropriate to say to someone, but it felt more like terror to his poor mom. She was understandably having a lot of trouble letting him go.

Additionally, Ryan's newfound independence was showing in many ways, both small and large. His musical tastes had left the world of Disney and had graduated to Michael Jackson (he still likes classic rock the best). The only time that he argued with his family to any extent was when he felt that he was being crowded or hovered over, and he was looking for new ways to take care of things himself. Nothing was off limits to him now, and kept trying new things. The rest of the family returned home one night to find him cooking a meal of hamburger steaks, salad and sweet potatoes for everyone. Shocked and thrilled by his new skills and independence, his mom said she hugged him and cried, "Oh, Ryan!" His response, typical of a thirteen-year-old, was a laconic, "What?" as if he had been doing it for years as he continued flipping the burgers.

One day after school Ryan came home with the news that he'd been asked to join the ice hockey team and needed a permission slip signed. As always, concerned for his safety, his mom asked "The special needs team?" It was in that moment that Ryan created my all-time favorite line from the kids. "NO!" he said, "I'M NOT SPECIAL!" That became his mantra and anytime the school or his family started coddling him he'd say the same thing, "I'm not special!" To this day, Ryan's ND and I use that line all the time between ourselves.

The biggest obstacle for Ryan right now seemed to be a tug of war with his mother. He wanted to grow up and experience new things; she was afraid of him getting hurt. I asked what kind of advice she had received from the psychotherapist I'd referred her to about this.

"She said to treat him like he's thirteen. Easier said than done." A lifetime of having to watch his every move was proving a challenging habit to stop. They both needed some time to catch up!

Since they had been on the Protocol for over four months now, Ryan was pretty adjusted to it. From time to time though, he really wanted some off-Protocol treats and was becoming more vocal about it. I suggested that she discuss it with him, the pros and cons, and then let him make a decision about it himself. This was the first time I ever gave this particular advice, but it certainly wasn't the last. This one simple thing will often change a kid, especially an older one, from feeling deprived to feeling empowered. One of my techniques is to tell the kids that they are not being deprived, but instead being a "Paleo Warrior." As typical, after an initial victory splurge into forbidden foods, Ryan started making his own wise food choices. No more arguments and no more "sneaking" of food after that foray. Case closed.

Follow-up:

In November of 2009 I discharged Ryan from needing monthly appointments. He is now on a Phase 3 Protocol, although they admit that it is not always terribly strict.

Ryan continues to improve. By September of 2011 he was very frustrated that the school would not take him out of the autism classes he no longer needs ("I'm not special!") and just let him continue mainstream. It's been quite the battle with the school system that at one point turned into a legal battle. His parents refused to give up on him and his best interests and they were victorious. Last time I saw him in person, Ryan had turned eighteen. He's 5'9" now and 150 pounds of solid ice hockey player. He's handsome, happy and healthy, although he did need a shave.

His mom is one of my favorite people for many reasons, but one is because she still keeps me in the loop. Most people (understandably) want to move on and forget anything was ever wrong, but she still gives me updates. As I said, I understand it, but I really love it when people clue me in on their child's progress. She has also tried to help my work as much as possible and had even given newspaper interviews to try to further educate people about the health benefits of the Protocol. I also admire her more than I can say for *never* giving up on her son. At three it was decided that he was supposed to live out his life in a group home; well, I wouldn't be surprised to learn that his "group home" will be a college dormitory!

Sometimes when she calls in, I get to hear another story about how well Ryan is doing. There are so many of them it's hard to choose just one, but I think this one is my favorite. When he was sixteen, they had a meeting scheduled with some school officials regarding his "autism status." When she started to park the car, he asked her to just drop him off because he wanted to handle the meeting himself. After a bit of back and forth, she finally agreed and dropped him alone at the curb of the building. Being the protective mother she is, she couldn't help herself and circled around to make sure that he was okay. Watching through the building window she saw him walk into the office, introduce himself, and shake hands with everyone before being seated. She immediately called me on her cell phone crying, "My son is becoming such a man!"

Yes he is. And my bet? I don't think he's done yet.

CASE STUDY 17

Mom: *"I'm just calling to gush!"*

Notes:

Dig really well —
Gain weight —
Talks about my topics now) —
No problems
Food allya's nearly gone
"His dig so fantastic I can't believe it!"

Name: Cooper P. (Male - phone only)

Age: 8
DX: Autism
Other diets: "Everything"
ND: Linda Kane

With all of the cases I see where the people seem to disappear after their children recover, I also get my fair share of these kinds of calls. **I am including Cooper's case because he and his family did the Protocol one-hundred percent without me and he still had dramatic results.** I really want you to understand that this is completely possible! I can't possibly see every child and I have thus far not been as successful as I hope to be in the future with getting other practitioners on board; we are, however, indeed making much progress in that area. The desire to make the Spectrum Balance® Protocol more easily available for interested families and practitioners is the main reason that my brother and I started the NoHarm Foundation and offer a free download of the SBP that continues to be used all over the world.

By the time I got this phone call from Cooper's mom, he had been on the Protocol for five months and his original issues had already resolved. When she informed me of this right at the top of the call, I was a bit perplexed. I was, of course, very happy to hear from her, but why did she set up a phone consultation? "He's doing so fantastic I can't believe it! I just had to call to gush!" Please, gush away, Mom!

In this line of work you meet many dedicated parents, but Cooper's mom is a parent whom I would call exceptionally dedicated to helping her son. Despite dealing with autism for most of Cooper's life, she was unwilling to throw in the towel and "accept" that he would always have problems. Cooper's parents had tried all the diets: GFCF, GAPS, SCD, rotation diets, elimination diets, etc., makes me dizzy just thinking about it! They had tried multiple therapies: light, sound, play, and luckily for Cooper, finding an excellent neurodevelopmentalist. And through Linda, they found the Spectrum Balance® Protocol.

Often when someone recommends the Protocol to parents, they think about it for a while. Maybe download it and look at it as a possibility for the future. I've had people tell me that it sat on their desk for over a year before they got around to it, or until they received multiple "chance" endorsements. Not Cooper's mom! Despite the fact that they'd already tried multiple diets without effect, she downloaded it immediately after Linda told her about it. She combed through the dozens of pages of scientific evidence validating its efficacy on the NoHarm Foundation website, and ordered the DVD I had made to help people who have no ability to see me. Next, she took everything out of the house that was not Protocol-friendly and dug into many of the Paleo recipe sites for new ideas.

When I asked her if it was a big change from how they were eating before, she laughed at me. "How we were eating which time? We've done so many diets I've lost track. This thing is a breeze compared to most of them." She said that it had never even entered her mind to not try it. She just wanted to do it right!

Keep in mind that the following descriptions of Cooper's symptoms are all prior to starting the Protocol. I never even knew he existed until they had already been relieved!

The developmental delays very early on had been what Cooper's diagnosis was based on, and then even at eight years old, he had very little speech. Because he displayed no understanding of conceptual thought, his speech had consisted only of a few words and no sentences, and his reading skills were nearly nonexistent. As you can imagine, this was very frustrating to him and his lack of coping skills reflected his discontent.

As is so often the case, in addition to the developmental issues he also had some troubling physical problems. His mom described his food allergies as "severe and multiple," and most probably as a side effect of this he was also significantly underweight and could not develop any muscle tone. At eight years old he had weighed only forty-nine pounds.

The number-one most common symptom I see when a person (child or adult) has high manganese is nightmares. For the lucky ones they are merely "busy" dreams; with long plot lines, lots of color, action, and detail. These are the kind of dreams where you wake up and feel like you've been chased all night. The unlucky ones seem to pull their worst case scenario from somewhere in the dark recesses of their brains. I have had kids of all ages (even the tiny ones) tell me about their ugly, frightening dreams that were full of demons, murder, blood, or wild animals. The most common of these is that there is something attacking them, sometimes even their own parents. Cooper was not one of the lucky ones. He was having frequent "horrific" nightmares.

I've said it before, and I'm saying it again. This school of thought that these ASD-affected kids are "just fine" and it's okay to "just let them be themselves"… I'm not buying it. If you had sat across a desk from as many kids as I have as they describe the world of fears and nightmares they had lived in, you wouldn't buy it either. In fact, you'd probably loathe that idea as much as I do. Whenever anyone says something like that to me, I think of the kids and their descriptions of their lives. They're not "fine."

Within a week or so on the Protocol, all these issues began to drop away. Fortunately for Cooper, the nightmares were the first to go. He had one or two in the first two weeks, and none since.

His speech had kicked in with a vengeance and Mom reported that he was now "talking, talking, talking like a parrot." Within two months he had graduated from words to sentences, and now to conceptual thought. "He's able to talk about topics and he can stay on track." As I have come to expect, as soon as he could express himself, the frustrations and accompanying anxious behavior disappeared. "He's happy and coping now. I can't believe it!" He had gone for an assessment with his ND and received a three-word report: "He's doing phenomenal!"

The last issue to go was his food allergies. At this five-month mark he was still having a few problems, but his mom described them as "nearly gone." A few months in with the new diet Cooper had a growth spurt that not only left him taller, but he was rapidly gaining both muscle tone and healthy weight.

Because he was so many years behind, Cooper had some catching up to do, but his mom had no doubt that he would do it and do it well. He was understanding everything anyone said to him now, he could express himself, his reading was quickly accelerating, and he was acting more age appropriate and mature by the day. All he needed now was time.

Before I could suggest it myself, Cooper's mother told me that they had made the decision to keep him on Phase 3 of the Protocol as a lifetime plan. "I know this is working and there's no way I'll give it up." I think that's an excellent idea. As she said, with relief evident in her voice, "I'm done searching. I'm staying with you and Linda."

We ended our extremely pleasant conversation with me complimenting her for her dedication to finding a way out for her son. You'd think that somewhere in the last eight years they would have given up, but they stuck it out and remained hopeful. It had been a long road for all of them, but in the end they had found their way home.

CASE STUDY 18

> Most alarming: behavior lately
> has always been ly easy going, slept well
> Around 18 months - 2: More defiant,
> had to do more discipline =
> Last 3 weeks or so: Been hav "rage
> episodes." Yet seem "Seizure like" =
> notey phases her, doesn't even notice by
> spanked = Screamy, kicking, crying
> Yesterday: 3 episodes before noon!?
> Pulling away from my affection - weird

Name: Grace C. (Female)

Age: 2.5
DX: Was currently being assessed, suspected Autism
Other diets: None

Although Grace's case is far from unusual, she is a good example of one of the most common hiccoughs that can occur during the course of being on the Protocol. If you've been on the Protocol for some time and it seems to plateau or "stall out" in some way, you sometimes need to become a bit of a detective. Little things can be important.

Up until the age of around eighteen months, Grace had always been a happy and easygoing baby. When she started to become a little more defiant, her parents wrote it off to her becoming more mature and beginning to want to make her own choices. However, this "defiance" very quickly began escalating beyond anything that could be explained away. For example, when she would start to cry, she could not be calmed by herself or anyone else and it would escalate to the point where it was a full-blown tantrum complete with crying, screaming, and kicking.

At the same time, Grace had suddenly stopped using any spoken language and was relying completely on yelling and crying to communicate what she wanted. This led to her parents to taking her to a speech pathologist for an assessment. Before even getting the results of his testing, the examiner had already told them that due to her "significant lack of verbal utterances" he was unable to even try to assess her articulation skills. Her mom was not surprised. Grace's younger, one-year-old sibling "talks more than she does" Mom sighed.

While all of her symptoms had been building for over a year, they had recently and suddenly taken on a new character. "The most alarming thing is her behavior in the last three weeks," her worried mom told me. "She's having rage episodes that look like seizures." I have seen a few of these in my office, and they do look very much like seizures. The kids will completely stiffen up, then kick, scream, bite, hit, spit, as if they can't control what their body is doing. They are actually frightening to watch because the kids could so easily hurt themselves or others when they're in this state. These new episodes were even more strange since Grace had never had them prior to the last three weeks, and they were occurring more and more often by the day. "Yesterday, she had three before noon," her dad said, looking at Grace sadly.

When people encounter a fit like this, it is often a knee-jerk reaction to simply think that the child is "just spoiled." This attitude has been very apparent in many of the grandparents (and a few others) who have sat disapprovingly in on some of my appointments. When I often would discuss Menefe Syndrome and its many manifestations it can have on behavior, I have heard a lot of derisive snorts from a grandparent who thinks, "the kid just needs more discipline." The sentence usually starts with, "In my day…" and unfurls from there. If you have a child who has tantrums or melt-downs, I'm sure you've heard many variations of this particular speech. In this case, discipline was not the issue, as proper parental discipline has always been a cornerstone with this young family, but even that wasn't working now. "Nothing fazes her at all," explained her harried mom. "Discipline, talking, spanking… nothing."

Prior to the last three weeks, physical affection was always the best and most successful tactic to calm Grace down. Although it didn't work every time it would sometimes have some effect. Now, it was just making it worse. "If you even try to touch her she jumps away and yells. She used to be so affectionate," Mom said wistfully.

It was hard for me to tell what Grace's parents were thinking at this point. As I've mentioned, I very rarely see both parents and when I do there are usually more questions and discussion than usual. In this case, the couple remained very quiet. When I gave them a copy of the Protocol food list, they just flipped through it without making any comments. After they finished looking through it I asked, "So, does that look like something you can do?" Mom sighed. "Yes." I waited, but she didn't go on. "Do you have any questions about it?" I asked? Sigh. "No."

At first I could not understand their laconic attitudes and seeming lack of interest. Not in all my years doing this have I had someone who didn't have one single question! But when I looked at Grace's Dad, it came to me. Mom was looking once again through the Protocol, but he was just sitting, hands dangling off his knees. The painful look in his eyes as he watched his daughter sitting on the floor told the true story. This wasn't disinterest; it was more like shell shock. It was plain to see by his example that this was a man who felt not only love but a sense of duty to protect and provide for his family. And right now, all he felt was helpless. They weren't disinterested; they were worn out.

As I gave them the information of what was required to start Phase 1 of the Protocol, they continued to be quiet and unresponsive. Instead of pushing them anymore today, I just told them to call if they had any questions. Mom nodded her head as they rose to leave, and sure enough I got the expected call full of questions two days later.

One-month progress report:

Far from the quiet and non-animated couple I had seen before, it was all smiles today; including a beamer from Grace! During our first appointment she had not made any eye contact, and had in fact stayed as far away from everyone as the confines of my office would allow. Today, she came around to my side of the desk, pointed at my computer screen and asked, "Can I see?" When I nodded my head, she proceeded to pull herself up onto my lap for a better view.

While she was still sitting in my lap, I jokingly asked, "So I guess the pulling away from affection thing is getting better, huh?" They laughed, and agreed. "We're starting to see the old Grace again. She's back to humming and singing too." As she climbed down off my lap, she held out the front of her cardigan she was wearing and informed me, "I put it on myself!" then went to sit on Dad's lap.

"So I guess the not being able to talk thing is getting better too, huh?" This was great. We'd only been in my office for about five minutes and we had already had a few good laughs. I much preferred it over the deafening silence of a month ago!

The seizure-like rage episodes that had sent them scrambling for answers had stopped after the fourth day of the Protocol and had not returned since. There were a few nights she had seemed like she may be ramping up for one, but they were able to talk her down. "It didn't look the same," recalled Mom. "It looked more like she was irritated not angry." I made a pointed note in her chart about this, because in many cases, especially with the really little ones, irritation

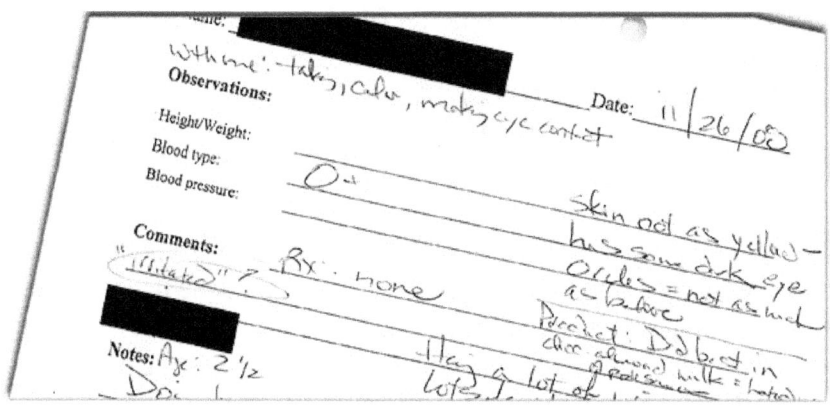

can be caused by pain that they don't have the capacity to explain. I'd keep an eye on that.

Getting the Protocol foods into her had been no problem. They were not fast food or junk food eaters anyway, so it wasn't even a huge change. In fact, little Grace had turned into one of the bottomless pits that I often hear about. Remarked her Dad, "Where does a two-year-old put half a meatloaf and three eggs?" Looking at the little snip of a girl sitting on his lap it did make you wonder.

Her speech had come on very suddenly, practically from one day to the next, about ten days into the Protocol. As her parents were leaving the house one morning she said, "Bye bye, Mommy. I love you, Daddy." Her words began coming quickly after that, and she was already starting to put them together in a more conceptual fashion. "She's started putting words together and being polite," bragged her Dad. Wanting to see if she knew what that meant, I asked her, "Are you polite Grace?" She replied,"Yes ma'am." Yep. She knew what I was talking about alright.

Since she was progressing so quickly, I told them that they could move onto Phase 2 of the diet, which allows additional foods. They went quiet again and exchanged a look. "Would it be okay if we just stayed on the Phase 1 we've been doing?" Mom asked. I told them that was no problem as she could feasibly stay on Phase 1 for her whole life and be healthy. They gave a relieved sigh at this. "You know what they say," said Dad, "if it ain't broke..."

Two-month progress report:

Despite the fact that I had only seen her a month ago, Grace looked noticeably larger, and I commented on that. "Yes, she had a growth spurt. The doctor said she's finally the right size for her age," Mom remarked. When she said this, Grace held her arms up and showed me that the sleeves of her sweater were now too short. "See?" she said proudly, "I'm big."

Although her rage episodes had not returned, she did experience one "very bad night" then was fine the next day. This is not unusual for kids on the Protocol, as they very often have a bad day or two and then make sizable gains afterward. When I asked for more details, Mom described, "It was so weird. It was like a wave came over her." First she got very irritated; nothing could please her, then she started to cry. They put her in the bathtub and she finally calmed down. Since it was an isolated incident and it happens so frequently I made a note about it but did not pursue it further.

Grace was once again becoming a joy to be around; very affectionate and sweet. "She loves to snuggle now and she gives big, good hugs" said Mom with a smile. While we were talking, Grace became very interested in some solar-powered dancing flowers I had on my windowsill. After watching them for a minute, she asked me if she could hold one if she was "very very careful." When I gave my permission she very gently took one down and watched it dance in her hand. Giggling, she gently placed it back in its place in the window. "Thank you," she smiled, then went back to sit with her parents. Many kids her age would have grabbed it without asking, but the politeness had seemed second nature to her. Apparently, gracious manners were coming on as fast as her speech.

In the prior month, Grace had gone from nearly silent to babbling happily, then speaking some sentences. Today, it was all sentences. During the entire appointment, she was talking away either to her parents or to me, using all full and expressional sentences. Like a lot of kids, she remembered my sticker collection and asked if she could go pick one out. When her parents and I came down the stairs she was deep in discussion with my receptionist as to whether she preferred the one with the flowers, or the one with the dinosaurs. I suggested she take both and her parents did not need to prompt the "Thank you" or the hug I got as a reward.

Three-month progress report:

With as well as Grace was doing I was surprised to see them this month. Generally, when children attain this level we just let it go a few months before checking back in. Things were not going badly, and her progress was not slipping, but something was unmistakably different.

Mom felt that her daughter had "hit a plateau" of some sort. It was hard to explain; she was not angry or violent, and her language was continuing to progress, she was just "off and weird." Questions about her diet told me that they had not had any off-Protocol foods, and that her appetite was still good. Flipping back through her chart, I noticed that I had circled the word "irritated" and added a question mark.

Starting with the most common causation I see, I asked Grace if her tummy ever hurt. Frowning, she nodded her head yes. "Can you show me where?" I asked. Standing up, she covered her belly button with her hand. I knew what that area indicated! Not wanting to complain, she had not told her mom that she was in pain. With my next question, "Is it hard to go potty on those days?" At this, Mom had a face-palm moment -- *of course!* She was constipated! Since Grace was potty trained she had not paid much attention to it. This should be an easy fix!

Further questioning revealed that the main cause of her constipation was most likely not enough healthy fats in her diet. Like many people, they were having a hard time getting over the "fat phobia" that most of us have, and as a result Grace's protein-to-fat ratio was off. Shaking his head, Dad admitted, "It just feels so weird to be putting butter and coconut oil on everything. I keep feeling like I should be guilty about it." I told them that most people feel that way but to take a look not only at Grace but themselves. She may have put healthy weight on, but they had both obviously taken weight off. Laughing, he repeated, "It just feels so weird!" His daughter then commented, "Yeah, Daddy, but it's yummy!" She's certainly right about that!

Four-month progress report:

With the good fats up, and the occasional help of an herbal tea, the constipation issue had resolved. The "off" days stopped and her progress, which had stagnated slightly, was moving forward again.

Replacing the rage she had once had was a gentleness and affection she had never shown. "It's so cute, she's mothering her brother now." They had been concerned a few weeks back when Grace warned that she was "going to throw a tantrum." Going to? Quickly they realized that she was using the threat of an imminent melt-down in an attempt to get her way! "She's very bright and I know she's using it now," said Mom, giving Grace the side-eye.

The kids who usually try this are older than Grace but it is extremely common. They spend their whole lives knowing that having a melt-down in the grocery store is a very effective tool to get their way, and they are loathe to give it up. It often takes a lot of discipline and discernment at this stage to coax them out of it. "Discipline we can handle," said Dad. "It was that other stuff that was freaking us out."

Because of her recent progress, Grace's parents had decided to get a new assessment of her skill levels. Their doctor had proclaimed, "Whatever you're doing, keep doing it," but displayed no interest in learning any details about the Protocol. This shocked them that he could see the progress with his own eyes, and even encouraged them to stay with it, but had no curiosity to learn more. Parents are always amazed, but it was 2009 by then and I was used to it. As "allopaths," conventional physicians, both general practitioners and most specialists, are not trained to focus on diet and nutrition as either cause or effect in their patients' conditions they are often not very interested in what the kids are eating. That's what naturopaths and nutritionists are here for since diet is the primary focus of what we study.

The lengthy assessment, which included occupational therapy, speech, and a psychologist, "blew them away." She was able to make many fine distinctions in her language, such as when asked if the tea was hot or cold, she responded that it was warm. My favorite was when the therapist showed her a picture of a dog and asked how she felt about dogs. She informed him, "That looks a lot more like a coyote to me." Spoken like a true daughter of the southwest! Although neither her parents or I could hear anything wrong with her speech, the examiner had suggested she see a speech therapist. She had started a week before this last appointment, and the therapist said she was "doing great."

Although I told her parents that a more standard Paleo diet would be fine for them now, they made the decision to stay on Phase 3 of the Protocol. The two are very close anyway, and well, better safe than sorry!

Follow-up:

I discharged Grace in March of 2009. I haven't heard from them lately but the people who referred them in told me she has continued to do just wonderfully.

She's such a funny little thing. During our last appointment when we all stood up to leave, she put her finger on the rather feminine belt I was wearing over my skirt. She said, "Look. Daddy has a belt on his outfit too." We all laughed, as his "outfit" and mine were quite different. As he looked down at her I remembered that look of helplessness I had seen in his eyes in that first appointment when he looked at her. What was in his eyes today was quite different. Today, it was unmistakably pride.

CASE STUDY 19

Mom: *"We had a parent-teacher conference and they said everything is terrific."*

Notes:
Age: 12

DX: Aspergers on Nov. 22, 07 = (date)
4 yrs. ago =
1/4 low focus =
Social = can't interact with older kids
Shuts down
had night terrors until age 6 or 7

Other DX: ADHD, Sensory Integration Disorder,
Depression

Name: Brandon W. (Male)

Age: 12
DX: Aspergers, ADHD, Sensory Integration Disorder, Depression
Other diets: None

Contrary to what the current paradigm believes, Brandon was one of the many kids I've seen who started out life perfectly fine. There is a pervasive belief system in the autism world that if you don't obtain that diagnosis by the age of two, there isn't going to be very much you can do to help them. **Brandon was one of the many who proves that theory flawed; as he wasn't even affected yet at that age.**

He was officially diagnosed at age eleven, but his symptoms had emerged and begun a downward progression four years earlier when he was seven. It started rather innocuously with his focus beginning to drift. School just seemed too noisy and distracting and his grades began to fall as a result. As this kind of thing is pretty common in kids his age, his parents weren't terribly concerned. However, as it often happens, it wasn't long until another issue cropped up. And then another. And yet another…

Soon after he began to lose his ability to focus, Brandon became extremely irritated by a wide variety of sensory input. First it was just school that was too noisy, then he could not stand to be in any kind of public place like a shopping mall or a movie theater. School assemblies and sporting events were definitely out since "applause drives him crazy."

Following this, his speech, which was always normal, became garbled and slow. It continued to worsen and by the time I met him he was barely intelligible. His mom said that he had "no social skills" and could not interact at all with other kids. From my perspective I have a tendency to think that this might have been, at least partially, embarrassment over his poor speech. Kids his age can be pretty brutal and it might have been easier for Brandon to simply avoid the situation.

Next, Brandon began to have intense skin sensitivity and he couldn't stand virtually anything touching him. Even clothing tags "drove him crazy." This presented itself in our appointment by his continual twitching, foot tapping, and constant standing up then sitting back down again. It was clear that the poor guy wasn't comfortable in his own skin. Although he was wearing a huge loose sweatshirt and big baggy basketball shorts he continually pulled and tugged at his clothes. You may be thinking that this kind of attire seems pretty normal for a twelve-year-old in most cases, but not in Colorado in January. Making the choice to freeze rather than let clothes touch him alerted me to the severity of the issue.

It was shortly before his official diagnosis that he finally manifested the one symptom that his parents could not ignore or dismiss as "personality" or "being a teenager." Brandon started "shutting down." All of a sudden and with no obvious trigger, it was like he wasn't there anymore. Talking to him, shaking him, nothing could make him snap out of it. It was frightening, and it was the final straw his parents needed to admit that something was definitely wrong.

There is no doubt in my mind that Brandon would have never ended up in my office if it were not for the person who referred them to me. It took almost a year of arm twisting from her just to get Brandon's mother to make the appointment for him. Although not openly hostile, which believe it or not people sometimes are, I would say his mom was very much in the skeptical camp. Although I always explain the science behind my approach, she asked me to explain it several times; each time giving me the same disbelieving scowl, a deep sigh, and flipping the pages of the copy of the Protocol.

My first approach with the more aggressive people, is to speak quietly and calmly and not be confrontational, but after about the third time I went through it, she actually waved a copy of the Protocol at me and challenged disbelievingly, "So this is it? He just eats this way and he gets better. That's it. That's what you're telling me." I explained (again) to her that there is of course, no guarantee, but that we had many years of success with it, and because it just involves eating healthy food there is absolutely no downside.

Another deep sigh and an exasperated look through the foods listed in the Protocol. She read, I waited, Brandon got up and down a few times and tugged at his sweatshirt some more. Again, she waved the document at me. "So just this? Food? He eats this and he might get better?"

A little done with repeating myself, I just smiled and confirmed, "That's the plan."

One-month progress report:

Over the next week, my office received a few phone calls regarding
the Protocol dietary guidelines from Brandon's mom. They were
pretty basic questions and were easily fielded by my staff, but I took
it as a good sign that she was trying to optimize to get the most she
could from having him on the Protocol.

As I've mentioned before, when you see extremely rapid progress
it's usually in the little kids; the one- to five-year-old set. Because
Brandon was twelve, taller than me, and weighed about 130 pounds,
I had warned Mom that it may take a little longer to see results, and
they needed to be on the look-out for the more subtle changes. Dang
kids. Always trying to prove me wrong.

When I went down to my waiting room to greet them for the second appointment, it was easy to see that some changes had already
occurred. Brandon, wearing weather-appropriate attire and a snow
jacket this time, gave me a big beaming smile and a friendly hello.
Even with that one word I could tell that his speech had improved.
Mom, formerly known as "the skeptic," couldn't wait to fill me in on
all the news.

They hadn't had to wait long to start to see results. Brandon's speech
had begun to clear after only one week on the Protocol, and now,
only one month in, it sounded perfectly normal. As I had suspected,
his garbled speech seemed to be linked to both his inability to social-
ize with other kids, and to his depression, since both had taken a definite turn for the better. After the second week on the Protocol, Brandon had started having conversations with the other kids at school,
and had joined the basketball team. He was still having issues with
one kid, but you know, there's just always that one guy, isn't there?

The irritating sensory issues, while not completely gone, were greatly
improved. The classroom didn't seem overly noisy now and he was

Name: ████████████████ **Date:** 3/4/08

Observations:

Height/Weight: _____

Blood type: O + _____

Blood pressure: _____

Comments: Ref: none

(Note: I noted his speech is very good)
(last 1/24/08 / ████ : Noticed how much speech changed
in one week)

Notes:

Doing really really well = "Mild mild hyper"
"Teachers are thrilled" New volunteer in class
Grades are coming up - he's getting
caught up: recently got an H on
a math test = not been sent to the
principles office at all
"It's so exciting to hear all good stuff"
Had a great teacher conference and
teacher said exactly this "terrific"
Diet: likes it for the most part "wishes wants"
Focus: much better - reading much better
Social/shutting down: No shut downs at all -
only an issue with one kid
Night Terrors: None - sleeps a bit better
Some input: still has irritation at times but
it's much less
Plays basketball @ school = Not happy his foot or
figety

Set Next Appointment Date? _____

205

feeling more able to focus. This improved focus was reflected by his reading and math scores going up to A's, and with all his grades steadily improving. Most remarkably, he had not had a single one of the "shut downs" that had sent his parents rushing for a diagnosis. Speaking for myself, I was glad to see him wearing weather-appropriate clothing and not flopping around in his seat like a stranded trout, and I was even more pleased to see him smiling. He was obviously much more comfortable in his body.

When I asked Brandon for his input, he said, "Overall, I'm much happier. I have my moments about the diet but I like it for the most part. It's definitely worth it." Pretty together for a twelve-year-old if you ask me.

As for Mom, she was thrilled about the changes in his school life. In the past, being called in for a parent-teacher conference was not exactly a rewarding concept, but now it was a whole different story. "It's so exciting to hear all good stuff! His teachers are thrilled! We had a parent-teacher conference and they said everything is terrific."

With all this exceptionally good news, I encouraged them to continue on to Phase 2 of the Protocol, and was looking forward to seeing what changes a second month would make in this young man. He just seemed so happy.

Follow-up:

It was a big decision on my part to give you the follow up's in some of these cases. Although all the kids all had a happy ending, it is not always so with me. In the name of complete honesty, which is what this book it about, here's what happened next.

Brandon was one of the "bittersweet" cases for me. When people find out what I do for a living, they almost all say the same thing, "Your work must be so rewarding!" For the most part they're right, it is exceedingly rewarding. But sometimes it is also tinged with other emotions for me. I am proud and thrilled for Brandon and that's the main thing, but I got a little dinged personally on this one.

On the day of his next appointment a month later, his mother called to cancel, saying that Brandon had a cold. She did not reschedule, and I never heard from her again.

Unfortunately, I've gotten rather used to this, since many who recover so well want to just move onward and upward and forget any past issues. However, this one wasn't quite done with me yet.

The person who referred them in is a long-time client of mine, and definitely very happy with the work I've done for her family. One morning, she called my office very upset. Apparently, she had run into Brandon's mother at the grocery store, and asked her how he was doing. After telling her that the school, their family, and everyone else was agreeing that Brandon was "perfect," my client asked, "And what does Shauna say?" Mom informed her that they didn't plan to go back to me because they "Didn't want to have to pay any more money."

My client continued to rant to me about what she felt was a travesty, but I must admit I went a little deaf at this point. I was envisioning the depressed, twitching, miserable boy who was failing at school and could barely speak, who, in only one month, became a happy guy who volunteers at school and is on the basketball team! The multiple diagnoses of Aspergers, ADHD, Sensory Integration Disorder, and Depression all a thing of the past! How much money was that worth? I tried to let it go, but my curiosity got the better of me.

So how much was "too much money?" Too much to come back? I pulled his chart and totaled up all his receipts. Including office visits and supplements it came to $667.58. Wow. I guess at least some part of his mother remained a skeptic.

That said, I absolutely do understand that some families are indeed in financial hardship mode, and being cash-strapped can occur for anyone at any time. I like to believe, however, that the cost of working with me and the Protocol is far less a hardship than the costs of doctors, drugs and medical treatments that may not fully bring a child back into the light of health, well being and happiness -- and a shot at having a great future. Or, let's put it another way, working the conventional way is a cost; working this way is an *investment*.

CASE STUDY 20

Mom: *"It's a night and day difference!"*

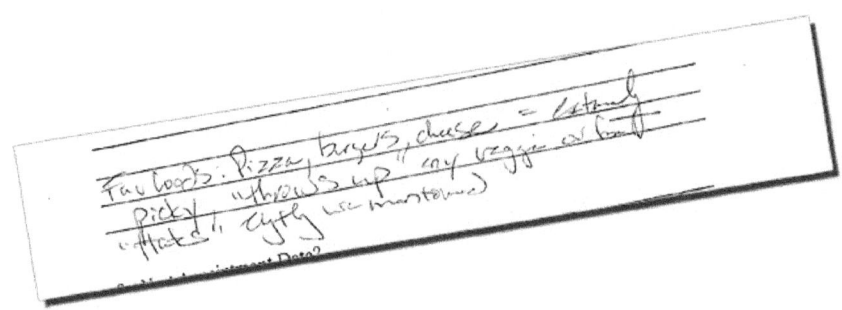

Name: Liam H. (Male)

Age: 7.5
DX: Separation anxiety
Other diets: None. "He only eats three foods"
RX: Albuterol

If you have ever heard the phrase "my child only eats…" come out of your mouth, then you definitely need to read this one. When I have personally heard that statement (and I have heard it a lot), it is generally followed by a litany of junk food that no one should be eating with any regularity if they want to be healthy. **No matter how strong their objections, kids will eat the food from the Protocol when they get hungry.** They may yell and scream, but they won't starve. It is up to the parents to make sure that the right foods are the only ones in the house, and they need to stand strong when the macaroni and cheese wars get started.

If it were not for his grandma, who is one of my long-time, diehard, "loves me" clients, I would never have seen Liam. She actually made the appointment, threw her daughter and grandson into the car, and drove them over 450 miles to my office. Sometime in that eight-hour drive, she must have gotten through, because by the time I saw them his mom was ready to talk to me.

Grandma had already given me the heads up that Liam's mom was "in denial." His physical issues, the ones she was concerned with, could have been easily taken care of by cleaning up his currently awful diet. His emotional issues on the other hand, although severe, were barely mentioned. Those were the ones that his grandma was most concerned with, but it was like pulling teeth to get any description of them from his mom. Liam and I had to sit through quite a battle between his mom and grandma to finally extract those details!

It was easy to see why they felt that the basis of his anxiety was all emotional. At only three years old, Liam's father, with whom he was very close, left a note saying he was "leaving and was never coming back." He was as good as his word and kept that "promise" -- the family had never received a single word from him in the following four and a half years. Understandably, this was devastating for Liam, but I believe his issues were caused more by what followed his father's disappearance than the actual event. Even when Mom re-married to a very nice man, Liam's anxiety continued to escalate. It had recently become so severe, and he was missing so many classes because of it, that they had been forced to take him out of school.

After his father left, his mother wanted to do as much as she could to try to make life easier for him, and unfortunately this included giving him anything he wanted to eat. This quickly turned into a lot of sugar, snack food, and junk food, until it reached the point that this junk was all he would eat.

His diet, if you could call what he was eating "food", was the biggest stumbling block in Mom's mind. On the drive to Colorado, his grandma had explained that my Protocol, while very effective, was all food related. Every time she would mention a food, Liam would sneer, "I hate that!" He continued to repeat this over and over during my appointment with him, so you could easily see the origins of her doubt.

When I asked what he did eat, it was a short list. "He'll only eat pizza, burgers and cheese." Nothing else. Liam added, rather defiantly, "I hate anything else. I won't eat it." Over time, he had developed a very clear way to demonstrate this "hate" by forcing himself to vomit if he was made to try anything off his list. All vegetables and fruits were on his "hate" list, and if he was coerced to take even the tiniest nibble of one, he would make himself throw up; an extreme but pretty effective tool to keep his parents from trying to get him to eat them!

The vomiting thing is interesting. It is amazing the tricks that kids can come up with to be able to get their own way. Although I've seen it more times than I can count, the parents all seem to think that their kid is the only one in the world who does it. I guess it's not something that you would care to bring up in conversation with anyone so it's not surprising. Just know that if your child does this, you are far from alone!

So with Liam either hating and/or throwing up anything that was good for him, what were we to do here? During our discussion of the Protocol, Liam began repeating "I'm gonna throw up, I'm gonna throw up…" like a disgusting chant. Just as I was getting ready to put an end to it, his grandmother spoke up. Looking at him sharply, she warned, "Liam. Knock it off!"

The puke chant thankfully stopped, but the whining and complaining did not. At the mention of the foods he would need to eat if he were to take on the Protocol, he intermittently cried, grabbed his face and moaned, purposely fell out of his chair, and made multiple mentions that he was "going to die." When he stood up and grabbed his mom's arm and flinging his arm out at me yelled, "Let's go! I hate her!" I'd had enough. Although I usually send the kids downstairs on an imaginary errand when I want to talk tough with their parents, this time I didn't. I wanted him to hear what I had to say in the hopes that it would reach him as well.

Over time I have learned that what children often truly want is to be perceived as more mature or grown up. If you've ever asked, "How old are you? Ten?" to a six-year-old and received a beaming smile in response, you know what I mean. This was the opposite of that equation. I asked him, "How old are you"? His whiny response was predictable, "Almost eight." Every kid to whom I've ever asked that question and who is close to "# and a half" always rounds up. My next question to Liam: "Do you think you're acting like an eight-year-old?" Blinking at me in confusion he didn't respond, so I asked the rest of the room. "Does anyone here think Liam is acting like an eight-year-old"? Now it was Mom's turn to cry. Her mother patted her on the shoulder in a comforting manner, but she also gave me the "go-ahead face" over her daughters shoulder. Grandma was definitely on my team.

After Mom calmed down, we had a very brass tacks discussion about food. I explained the very simple fact that when Liam got hungry, he would eat. Period. He would not starve by missing a meal, or even a few meals. I told her about one case I had where a five-year-old girl went five days without eating; in fact she threw all the food off the table. But, just like anyone, she finally got hungry enough on the sixth day to eat and it was all uphill from there. Liam's mother still obviously had her doubts, so Grandma intervened. "Look. I will come over to your house, we'll clean everything out that doesn't belong, then we'll go shopping. And I'll help you cook. Deal?" This was an offer she couldn't refuse, so she agreed.

Usually, when an appointment goes like this I don't have much faith in a good outcome. This time however, I had hope. I had a secret weapon -- Grandma.

One-month follow-up (phone):

As soon as they got home, Grandma made good on her word. Everything that wasn't Protocol-compliant got packed up and taken out. Liam, who never thought Mom would actually do it, increased the level and intensity of his protests, complaining that he was "being tortured," among other things. His protests fell on deaf ears for both his grandma and stepdad, and Mom resolved to steel herself to it, so the battle was on.

For the first few days, Liam pulled out all the stops. Crying, tantrums, dramatically proclaiming that he was "dying," that they were "terrible and hated him," and of course, his big gun, fake vomiting and gagging. Since it became clear after a few days that they were not going to give in to his demands, he predictably got hungry and resentfully started eating. Things improved quickly from that point on.

Within a few days, they were seeing marked changes in both his allergies and his anxiety. His allergies, which had been terrible ever since he had been weaned off breast milk at eighteen months, were very nearly gone. "His nose used to be like a faucet before, and now he barely has any."

As glad as they were that he was relieved of his allergies (and asthma, too), Mom was now willing to talk about his anxiety problems. When I asked her about it she gushed, "I'm so excited! He's doing so much better. I can tell such a big difference." His incessant wor-

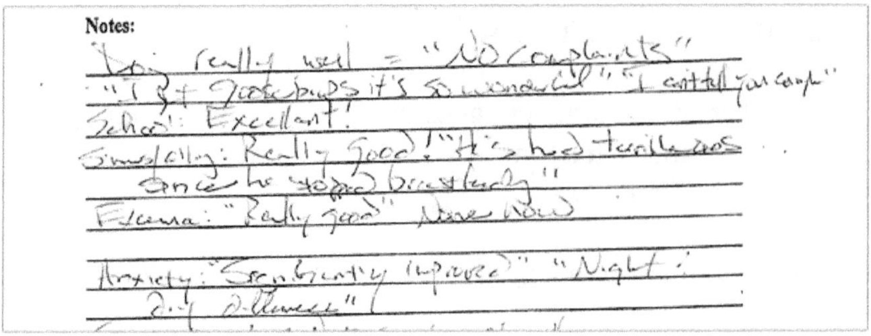
Notes:
Doing really well = "No complaints"
"I got goosebumps it's so wonderful" "I can't tell you enough"
School: Excellent!
Socially: Really good! "He's had terrible ... since he stopped breastfeeding"
Eczema: "Really good" None now
Anxiety: "Significantly improved" "Night and day difference"

rying over every minute detail, something he had done for years, was the first to go. After that he so steadily improved that they were able to put him back in school! "He still gets a little anxious with transitions, but it's so much better."

As far as the food on the Protocol, to her surprise, they were doing fine. Apparently after he waged his three-day battle campaign, he took well to his capitulation. While still being somewhat limited in what he liked, with veggies being the main issue, Liam was eating well with a good appetite. Even though his list of favorites was small, he was no longer "hating" foods and as his mom happily reported, "The fake pukes are gone. Thankfully." He would sometimes balk a bit at new foods, but he wasn't whining anymore.

The Protocol had started out being difficult, as it was quite a significant change; omitting a total junk food diet and replacing it with a high-nutrition diet so drastically is often the most difficult part for anyone. Fortunately, her husband had been willing to try it, and was very supportive of cleaning the non-compliant foods out of the house. But as I had predicted, it had been my secret weapon who carried the day. "I don't know what I would have done if it wasn't for my mom. She had to hold my hand at first." Being that Grandma is a several year veteran of Paleo eating, helping her daughter with the Protocol had been a breeze for her.

Since Liam was doing so well, I suggested that they stay on Phase 2 of the Protocol, and that we would touch base again in two months.

Two months later, Three months on SBP (phone):

Apparently, things were still on the upswing for Liam. His mother opened the conversation by exclaiming, "I can't tell you enough. I can't tell you fast enough! I get goosebumps it's so wonderful!" Now that's my idea of how to open a great conversation!

Since just after week-one of the Protocol, when they were beginning to notice the first changes, Liam's progress had not ceased. The allergies he had since he was an infant just tapered off then stopped. The eczema faded away shortly thereafter. But the biggest change was in the boy himself.

The crippling anxiety that had ruled his life was finally gone. As a result, his world was changing and he was showing it in many subtle ways. Going from only eating three foods only three months ago, his palate was definitely expanding. He would at least try most anything that was put in front of him (without pretending to vomit), and he was growing interested in foods he had not tried yet. To encourage this exploration, he and his grandma had even started perusing some Paleo recipe websites together.

He was happy at school and was getting "excellent" reports on both his behavior and his grades. He was sleeping better and would sometimes play in his room by himself now, something he was too paranoid and anxious to do before. "It's amazing. It's a night-and-day difference," beamed his mom.

When I asked her if there were any issues left to deal with, her immediate answer was, "Nope. Not a thing. I have no complaints."

As I always do when I'm getting ready to discharge a client, I gave her the speech about the dangers of sliding back into their old way of eating. Halfway through, she started to laugh. "Oh you don't have to worry about that. My mom would kill me!" Too true.

Before we got off the phone, I asked her to convey to Liam for me that I was really proud of him for doing so well on the Protocol, and for sticking with it himself at school. It reminded her to mention to me, "Oh yeah. Liam wanted me to tell you something too. He said to tell you he's acting eight now." It's funny, I wasn't even sure if he had really heard me when I said that, but apparently it had stuck with him. You just never know!

Follow-up:

Because he's doing so well, I don't hear from the them much, but I do speak with his grandma regularly and she says he's doing just great. I believe her because I'd surely hear about it from her if he wasn't! She has spoken many times about how glad she is that she "dragged my daughter in by the hair" to see me. She's not a big one for compliments, but I had to tell her how important I felt her participation had been. I don't believe they could have stuck it out without her, and I was very grateful for Liam's sake.

Her laconic reply is so typical of her. She just said, "Oh, I've been trying to get them Paleo for years. I'm just getting what I want out of the deal." Now that's a win-win if I ever encountered one!

CHAPTER EIGHT

Achieving Success with The Spectrum Balance® Protocol

Okay, let's demystify the entire process and dilute it to the basics. Here, in a nutshell, is the best way to achieve success using the Spectrum Balance® Protocol:

1. The entire family needs to do the Protocol together. Not only to get the wrong foods out of the hands of your kids, but to eliminate their desire for these foods because they can still see other family members eating them. If they can't see them, they'll forget about them.

2. **You must adhere to the Protocol strictly to get results. In the mass majority of cases, even 90% compliance will yield 0% percent result!! This cannot be stressed enough!**

3. Stay on the "Best" choices food list as much as you possibly can for at least the first sixty to ninety days. Too many foods from the "moderate" category during this critical phase can slow or possibly stop progress.

4. Watch for changes of any kind. Any behavioral change, even one that appears "negative" like tantrums or frustration, constitutes a reason to stick with it! ANY change at this point is positive! **The only negative is no change at all.**

5. Do what you can to get grass-fed, organic meats, butter, etc. but many times you'll have to do the best you can with what you've got. I've seen folks with very little budget for food, or in areas with limited availability of grocery stores, do extremely well with this Protocol.

6. Be positive! Use the approach of saying how yummy and good the food is and not dwell on what they aren't eating. Let the kids help decide and even help cook what they want to eat out of the allowed choices of the Protocol.

7. Get tough! Often the downfall of this is people outside the home or even family members who persist in the "a little won't hurt" mindset. I have had parents who had to keep their children away from family members who continually spoiled their progress because of this until the child completed the Protocol and was balanced.

8. Knock off the baked goodies. Because of the explosion of the Paleo lifestyle, there are thousands of recipes using "allowed" flours and there is a tendency to go nutty with the cookies and treats. **This slows or stalls the progress every time,** so save the allowable treats for special occasions. Yes, Mikey may not get his *regular* birthday cake this year, but isn't it worth it if you don't have to worry about food setting him off next year? Please don't allow holidays and vacations to ruin your child's progress.

9. Urge your child to speak. If he or she has been signing and/ or pointing for a length of time this won't change unless you take the reins. Create new habits! Make them use their words to get what they want!

10. Utilize the plethora of Paleo diet recipe sites. These meals can often be used with no or very minimal changes. Use the term "Paleo" first in the search bar as it will weed out any recipes

with grains; as in "Paleo (lasagna, chili, burgers, meatloaf, etc) recipes." To this purpose, I just now took a mini-break to do a Google search on "Paleo Mac & Cheese" and got 192,000 hits! Just make sure to cross check with your list of Protocol "avoid" foods and make sure none of those sneak in.

Also worth mentioning are a short list of circumstances that I have seen interfere with the Protocol being completely effective. Some of these you can do something about, and some you can't. However, they are all worth your consideration:

1. Trying to do too many things all at once. This is a big one. Often when people first go on the Protocol they are also on large regimens of supplements or other kinds of "therapies." This can easily turn out to be too much of a good thing! Concentrate primarily on the food for the first two to three months. That way there is no interference and you can tell what is working.

2. Trying to avoid cooking. Sorry, folks, but there really is no way around this. Anything ready-made or packaged is likely going to contain something that shouldn't be there. No two ways about it - you have to cook! And have the kids load the dish-washer...

3. Strangely extreme resistance from family and friends. Be ready for it! If you're already eating Paleo you probably know what I mean. If you're not, brace yourself. Why anyone else would care so much what you're eating remains a mystery to me, but it is definitely an issue. Promise yourself that you'll stick to your guns. After all, this way of eating will benefit your life too!

4. Resistance from your current doctors and/or therapists. It doesn't happen every time, but when it does it can be quite dramatic. There have even been a few specialists who refused to work with the child unless they stopped the Protocol, even

after they had seen positive and sometimes dramatic changes as a result of them being on it. Far be it from me to tell you who to work with, but I believe that any specialist with an open mind is going to be much more helpful and on board with your goal of your child's wellness than one who operates from "know it all" ego.

5. Do everything you can to avoid GMO (genetically modified) foods! In simplest terms, a GMO is a crop that has been genetically modified to produce a desired trait it currently doesn't have, such as being insect resistant. Although foods like soy and corn are disallowed on the Protocol anyway, there is more and more use of GMO's in tomatoes, papaya, and squash which are allowed. Do your best to buy organic for those products!

So, is this a big huge enormous change? I would say that for most people it is, but it is a vital change for you and especially for your kids! I had a mother who told me that her three-year-old son would only eat five foods: macaroni and cheese, pinto beans, peanut butter and jelly sandwiches, frozen waffles, and ramen noodles. That's it. She didn't feel that she could change that eating pattern because her child threw tantrums when anything else was offered, and it would be too difficult to overcome. How could anyone expect that a child could experience any level of current or future health and happiness eating like that? So sorry, but convenience foods and drive-throughs are pretty much out with this, for now anyway. Because of the enormous popularity of the Paleo movement there are many more new and wonderful convenient choices becoming available every day. So who knows; maybe soon we'll have a Caveman drive-through!

As with anything that creates lasting positive change, this will be a transition. Hopefully, these simple guidelines provided in this book will help to make it an easier and more fun transition for you.

It bears repeating -- the most important guideline of all is that Golden Rule: **In the mass majority of cases, even 90% compliance will yield 0% result!**

As long as you keep that one rule in mind, you're almost there.

21 - 25

In my over thirteen years of practice, one thing I have repeatedly heard from my clients is that they appreciate the fact that I never give up on them. This goes double and triple for me when it comes to these autism cases. No matter how steeply the deck seems stacked against them, in my world there is always hope.

Some of the cases I've seen did indeed seem hopeless. I've seen kids who were apparently vaccine damaged. Kids who were in their teens and beyond who were no longer considered "young enough" to recover. Many who were from hard home situations; children of divorce, abuse or abandonment. Some who had genetic or metabolic abnormalities that were thought to be insurmountable. Those whose futures looked bleak and empty with nothing but institutions, group homes, or possibly even prison to look forward to. It is absolutely amazing how many kids that were "going nowhere" have now arrived at their "somewhere" thanks to the Spectrum Balance® Protocol. Somewhere they actually wanted to be.

Because of this work I do, I am often asked if I have children, and I always give the same answer. "Yes I do. About three thousand of them". Although all "my kids" are precious and unique to me, somehow the ones that no one thought had a shot; that were "too damaged", or that I thought I'd never see again, hold a special place in my life.

These children - these lives - are not forfeit! Don't fall for that! So many are told that they are too old, or too severe, or too damaged in some fashion, but those reasons are not compelling enough to me to give up. Have you got one more big college try in you? I hope so...

Remember - The Spectrum Balance® Protocol is just food. The only downside you may encounter is more shopping and dirty dishes! After reading these remarkable case studies, I hope you feel that is worth a try.

CASE STUDY 21

Mom: *"We went from no hope to boatloads of hope. He has a bright future now."*

This is the only case study where we are using a real name. It is being used by permission as he used his real name previously in this video.

Note: You can see an amazing eight-minute segment from the television show EcoSense featuring Nick's story. Put "Assertive Wellness" into the search bar on YouTube, and watch "Dr. Shauna Young's television experience on "Eco Sense".

Name: Nick P. (Male)

Age: 6
DX: Autism, Bi-Polar Disorder, Oppositional Defiance Disorder, ADHD, Obsessive Compulsive Disorder
Other diets: GFCF prior, GAPS currently
RX: Lamictal, Zyprexa, Intuniv, Paxil, Tenex and Desmopressin
ND: Linda Kane

Many people who contact me about their children feel that they are at the end of their rope. This had become so common that a friend of mine (half) jokingly suggested I put in a pool and call my clinic "The Last Resort." But in July of 2010, I received a desperate email from a mom who truly was out of options. It would begin the most complex and the most rewarding case I have ever had.

There is a saying that you are never given more than you can handle, but I think poor Nick not only got his own problems but a few other people's as well. Born at thirty weeks to a mother who did not want him, even the circumstances of his birth were harsh. I am only thankful to whatever angels were watching out for him and brought him to his adoptive family. They are truly some of the most loving and amazing people I have ever met.

From his first day of life, Nick was "agitated." They could tell right away that something was not right with him, and by the time he was scarcely three months old there was no doubt. He was not developing the way a baby should at that age, and already, he was always angry. Even his digestion was impaired and the poor guy never had a single formed bowel movement until he was put on the GFCF diet many years later.

As if these struggles were not enough, at age three, disaster struck and Nick was hospitalized with meningitis/encephalopathy. Because of the inflammation in his brain, he began suffering seizures and went into a coma for more than a week. When he awoke, he had lost all bodily function. As his mom described, "He lost the ability to do anything but breathe."

After transferring him to a children's rehab hospital, Nick spent the next month relearning how to swallow, crawl, walk and talk. He was discharged on Lamictal, the first of his onslaught of drugs, for his seizures that had wracked his body while he was sick. The car ride home from the hospital however, proved that their troubles were far from over. When they put Nick in his car seat he began screaming. He said he felt "stuck" and "didn't want to be stuck." He screamed for the entire four-hour car trip.

From there, things just continued to grow worse. His anger was now morphing into violence; hitting, kicking and biting were all common. He was constantly making threats to kill himself and others, and he started repeatedly butting his head through the drywall in their home. He could no longer be taken out of the house at all and was requiring 24/7 supervision. The diagnosis and the prescriptions began to pile up in the attempt to modify or control his irrational and frightening behavior. He was lost, and his mother and sister decided the only option left was to get him in the car and drive him over 1,300 miles to see me on the recommendation of his ND.

When writing, you try not to use the same word over and over again to describe a situation, but in Nick's case, by the time I met him there was only one word to describe him. Extreme.

Extremely violent. Multiple times during our initial one-hour appointment he threatened to kill both me and himself. Listening to those threats coming out of a little kid that was so cute it made your teeth hurt was… impossible to explain. Extremely paranoid, especially of open spaces, overhangs, hallways and tall buildings. He was terrified to go into their own garage. It drove him to constantly ask his family if they were mad at him. Extreme noise sensitivity. Extreme nightmares and hallucinations that even his anti-psychotic medication had barely touched.

Without the medications, Nick was uncontrollable. The problem was, they were starting to cause problems of their own. The doctors had no answers, and it appeared that some form of institutionalization was the only option left to Nick.

So here they were, trying one last thing. The Protocol looked simple to his mother as it was quite close to how they were eating anyway. She accepted it with very few questions and a determination to give it a one-hundred percent try. She didn't care how it worked, she just needed it to work. There was nothing else left to try for Nick. To be one hundred percent honest with her, I told her that I had never worked with a child as extreme as Nick (she gave a tired laugh at that), and I had no idea if it could help, but I was more than willing to try. Mom nodded her head in understanding and said, "Well, it's just food so at least we know it won't hurt."

After they left my office to begin another 1,300-mile drive home, I sat thinking about what I had just seen. In the course of the years in my work I have met thousands of people, yet not one affected me like Nick. His life just seemed so unfair to me. Only six years old and living such a tortured life of fears and anger. Yes, listening to the death threats coming from his angelic face was chilling, but overall it was more heartbreaking. I prayed that the Protocol would help him.

Two weeks: (voice mail)

I came into the office one Tuesday morning, pressed a button and heard this: *"It's working! The violence has stopped. His paranoia is less. It's working!"*

I didn't even have to look to see who the message was from.

Over the next three months:

From here, instead of me telling you how it happened, I'm going to let Nick's mother tell it. I will tell you that his progress started in the first two weeks and continued to move steadily from there. The text below was a post to an SBP support group.

11/05/2010

We will be at three months on the diet on the ninth, so I thought I would post an update.

My son is completely Rx-free now! He was on anti-seizure, mood stabilizer, anti-psychotic, anti-depressant, and sleep medications when we started this SBP protocol. We had a honeymoon period with the diet the first month and then had to start weaning off one of his meds because of his A1c level being elevated. This caused an imbalance with another med which we then had to drop. He had horrific drug withdrawals from that.

I was ready to quit and just do the diet with drugs, but I couldn't because of the A1c level, so I took a huge plunge and started weaning all the meds one at a time while he was still going through the withdrawal from the worst one. Dr. Shauna had told me when the diet was first working for us that since it was working so well, she believed it would work completely. Weeks went by where I held on to her belief because all I had was despair, but my son has been drug free for three weeks now. This is the first time in three years that he has been off an anti-psychotic without seeing spiders or mice crawling on him. He is sleeping without sleep meds and not having nightmares.

Three days this week he has visited the tiny Christian school where my daughter teaches. She has a K / 1 split class with only six children, and the principal has given permission for my son to join in for music, P.E., recess, and non-structured center time. He did have a big ugly three-year-old style temper tantrum when we had to leave the first day, but this has not happened since. The building where the music class is has several overhangs, high open spaces, and long hallways, all of which are recipes for extreme panic and violent behavior no matter how much he wants to do something. He hid behind me a few times as we transitioned into these areas, then peeked around and came back up beside me and walked with me. It was as though he was anticipating horror, but it wasn't there.

We are working on the behavior program our Neurodevelopmentalist gave us the very first time we had an evaluation. It is so effective now that the complete panic/ rage/ other irrational emotions are gone. He does still have quite the temper, but there is at least a reason when he gets angry (even though the reaction is usually way larger than the cause). I do believe he has the capacity to learn self-control now, when before, I thought his future held some form of institution-alization.

I know my son's issues are different than those of most other kids, but I hope his story is an encouragement to you all. Thank you for all your help and prayers.

Four months:

Because Nick was doing so well, I was not talking to his Mom very often, and usually just a quick "he's doing great." At Christmas I received an email from her containing a link to a home video in which Nick was singing in the children's church choir for a Christmas pageant. He followed that up with a two-man stand-up comedy routine with another boy. I watched it five times.

Nine months: (email from his mom)

Hi all,

We were gone for the weekend and my adult daughters took the younger ones to Six Flags for the weekend. Nick got to go! He had a great time and was very well behaved! They cooked the day before they left and took all his food with them. On Sunday they sent me the following message. It really did this mom's heart good. Last year there would have been no way he could have made this trip, much less happily. I'm so excited for his present and his future.

So Nick didn't eat much tonight. I tried to convince him and he said, "I can't, my stomach is too filled up with joy."
Sent from my iPhone

Follow-up:

As I write this, Nick is almost eleven. Of their choice, the family members still follow the Spectrum Balance Protocol. I told them that they could go off it and onto a regular Paleo diet, but they decided to stick with it. I guess when your son was butting his head through walls and hallucinating that mice were crawling on him you have more of a desire to stick with what works.

When I visited their home a few years back to film the EcoSense episode, Nick answered the door. I asked if he remembered me, and like any other kid his age he rolled his eyes at me. "Duh! We talk about you all the time." I did get a hug though, so I let the eye rolling go.

Looking at the patched places on the walls, it really hit home for me what these people had endured. Hearing about a kid bashing his head through drywall is very different from looking at the massive holes that had been repaired. Now he was just a happy, healthy kid, with a wicked sense of humor.

While being shown around their house, I suppose I got kind of quiet, because his mother asked if anything was wrong. No, nothing was wrong, it was just all so right! I always have been (and probably always will be) emotional when it comes to Nick. Although I am grateful for the recovery of all my kids, I guess I just have some extra gratitude when it comes to Nick. By that very moment, as I stood in their living room, he would have most likely already spent several years in an institution. His path had been so dark, and now it was full of shining light.

When I told his mom about this overwhelming sense of gratitude I had surrounding Nick, she looked at him, currently zooming around the kitchen with a red towel over his shoulders in his best superhero imitation. "Nick was in such devastating circumstances. I didn't know what his future would be. He has a bright future now."

Yes, he does. The deck was well and truly stacked against Nick right from the beginning; thank goodness his mother was unwilling to let it stay that way. God bless families like this.

Although Nick's story is compelling, amazing, awesome, what I most feel is gratitude. How do you express what it was like to be a part of this... this miracle that happened for such a deserving child? I'm just so grateful that I was fortunate enough to be a part of his story.

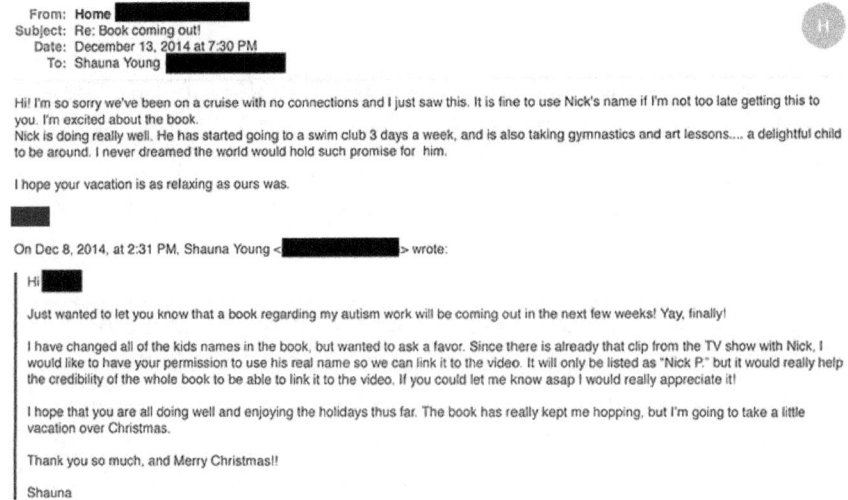

From: **Home**
Subject: Re: Book coming out!
Date: December 13, 2014 at 7:30 PM
To: Shauna Young

Hi! I'm so sorry we've been on a cruise with no connections and I just saw this. It is fine to use Nick's name if I'm not too late getting this to you. I'm excited about the book.
Nick is doing really well. He has started going to a swim club 3 days a week, and is also taking gymnastics and art lessons.... a delightful child to be around. I never dreamed the world would hold such promise for him.

I hope your vacation is as relaxing as ours was.

On Dec 8, 2014, at 2:31 PM, Shauna Young < > wrote:

Hi

Just wanted to let you know that a book regarding my autism work will be coming out in the next few weeks! Yay, finally!

I have changed all of the kids names in the book, but wanted to ask a favor. Since there is already that clip from the TV show with Nick, I would like to have your permission to use his real name so we can link it to the video. It will only be listed as "Nick P." but it would really help the credibility of the whole book to be able to link it to the video. If you could let me know asap I would really appreciate it!

I hope that you are all doing well and enjoying the holidays thus far. The book has really kept me hopping, but I'm going to take a little vacation over Christmas.

Thank you so much, and Merry Christmas!!

Shauna

CASE STUDY 22

Mom: *"I feel like he's just getting up the courage to turn 17 and kill himself."*

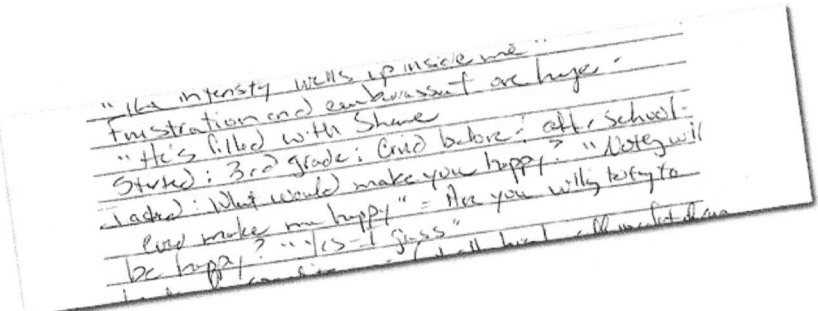

Name: Quinn T. (Male)

Age: 11
DX: Mood Disorder
Other diets: Raised on soy baby formula

Has been seen by multiple MDs and naturopaths. Sees a psychiatrist twice a week.

Although this is not an "autism" case, I felt it was important to include it. **There are so many kids like Quinn out there who are unreasonably unhappy for no reason their parents can figure out, and usually the only solution offered is medication.** Even the naturopaths that they had tried had reached for a Band-Aid that would treat his symptoms rather than looking for the cause. A GABA combo and 5-HTP had helped a bit, but he was still, and ever increasingly, miserable.

In all my years in practice, I have never met a person, adult or child, who was more just plain sad than Quinn. At an age where he should be out having fun with his friends, his world consisted of constant anxiety, isolation, shame, depression, and thoughts of suicide. Despite nearly constant medical intervention it had become so severe over the years that now he couldn't even go to school. "I want to" he told me, "but I know I can't. I'm a bad person."

Talk about a Hail Mary pass by his mom. By now Quinn was seeing a psychiatrist twice a week who was adamant about prescribing the boy a cocktail of psychiatric medications; something his mom was vehemently opposed to. She knew the Protocol was going to be a hard sell in her family, but she was willing to try anything. Her husband was 100% opposed to any kind of "weird diet," and Quinn was so depressed and enveloped in feelings of hopelessness and apathy she knew it might be harder to get him to comply. I felt she was hoping that I might be able to talk him into it, so I spent more of the appointment speaking directly with Quinn than with his mom. When kids are this age I have found that the more I hold them personally responsible the better the results.

"The last thing I want to do is drug him" said his frustrated mother, "but we don't know what to do. He doesn't enjoy his life and he's filled with shame."

It wasn't hard to treat Quinn like an adult. Obviously highly intelligent and extremely articulate it did not seem at all like a conversation with a child. In fact, he bordered on being too articulate when describing the prison his own mind had become. I listened professionally, but inside all I wanted to do is get up and hug the poor kid, which is not a good move when you're trying to treat him as more of a grown-up.

When I asked him where he thought the source of all this unhappiness was coming from, he said in his eloquent fashion that he felt it was stemming from a feeling of "intensity" that he could not control. "The intensity wells up inside me until I feel like I'm going to explode." He avoided any kind of contact with people because even the slightest comment from someone that he could perceive as critical would bring on crushing feelings of embarrassment. He told me that he had frequent and terrible nightmares, but would not divulge what they were about. "I'm too embarrassed by them. Embarrassment and frustration are huge in my life."

While I was discussing the specifics of the Protocol with them, Quinn continued looking down at his lap. When I would ask him directly if he understood something I said, he mostly responded with either a lethargic nod or a shrug. It is simply a fact that when kids his age don't want to comply with the diet, you can't force them. They can always either buy their own junk food, or get it at school or a friend's house -- there are plenty of sources. The added complication of his dad not being on board pretty much assured me that there would be plenty of non-Protocol-compliant foods right there in the house. I needed to get Quinn engaged and on board.

"Quinn, think about this; what would make you happy?" After pondering for a moment and without lifting his head, he replied, "Nothing. Nothing will ever make me happy." I decided to take a shot. With a more steely tone, I commanded, "Quinn, look at me." Apathetically, he lifted his head and made his first real eye contact with me. "There is a chance that this Protocol could make you feel better, but it won't work if you don't want it to. Are you willing to try to be happy? Will you try?" A light seemed to come on in him. At first he looked puzzled, and then I got a half smile out of him. "You're pretty weird. No one has ever asked me that before. I guess I could try."

As we all stood up to leave the office after the appointment, Quinn turned at the door. Looking me in the eye again he said, "There are a lot of mean people in this world. I wish they were all dead!" and then turned to walk down the stairs. I stood there for a moment fervently hoping that he didn't think I was one of those meanies.

I doubted I would ever see them again, but I was wrong.

<u>One-month progress report:</u>

As soon as I saw them in the waiting room, I knew there had to have been some change. Sitting with them on the couch in the waiting room was Dad, who had been completely resistant to his son and wife seeing me in the first place. When I was shaking his hand I told him that it was nice to see a father there, as I usually just work with the moms. He admitted to having been against the whole thing right from the beginning, and I complimented him for being open minded enough to change his opinion. "I needed to see proof" he stated, "now I have it."

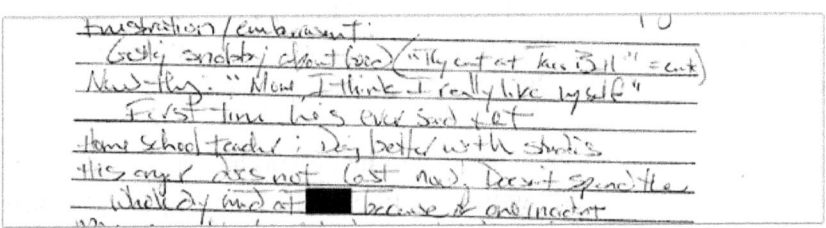

Right from the beginning they started seeing consistent change in Quinn. As it turns out, he and his dad had a very prickly relationship for some time and they saw a nearly immediate difference there. When his father had recently asked him to do a chore, he got a compliant, "Okay, Dad!" instead of his usual arguments. "That was a first," reported Dad.

His anger in general was lessening in severity. As his mom explained, "When he gets mad it doesn't last and he comes to logical conclusions." There were significantly fewer confrontations and for the first time in Quinn's life he was displaying a willingness to cooperate.

Thankfully the "intense" feeling Quinn had been unable to completely describe had let up as well, and the nightmares had stopped. As a result the anxiety, depression and mood swings were occurring less frequently and with greatly decreased intensity. He was more able to relax and was opening up to new experiences. He had even been able to join the family to see a program at his sister's school. When his mom discussed this outing, she noted that Quinn had smiled and commented, "They all eat Taco Bell at that school. Lame!" Okay, so he was also becoming a food snob. I can live with that.

With all this good news, there was one major snag. When his psychiatrist noticed how much better he was doing, Quinn's mother excitedly told him about the Protocol he was on. Upon hearing this, the doctor "exploded." He was so incensed, he thoroughly denounced both them and me, with the upshot being that he refused to even see Quinn unless his parents allowed him to immediately put the boy on the medications he prescribed and took him off the Protocol. Needless to say, they don't see him anymore.

Unlike the first appointment, this time, Quinn was much more animated and engaged, and I suddenly noticed what a handsome boy he was when he smiled. He was actively participating in the conversation and was asking questions about various foods that he liked or disliked, and of course, how long he would have to be on the Protocol. I told him that he would most likely have to be strict on it for several months, and after getting off it he still could not return to eating as he had before. He thought about it and asked, "If I did, could all of this come back?" I told him that yes, that was a distinct possibility. He made a quick decision on that one! He immediately said, "Not gonna do that then," with a dismissive wave. I suggested he do some reading about Paleo to get the ground work. He heartily agreed and decided to start with "The Paleo Solution," since he liked the exercise information as well.

Although there had been no recent talk of suicide, I asked him to be completely honest in how he felt about it. He admitted that there were "some tiny bits of it," left but it was not the all-encompassing issue that it had been before. He agreed with me when I suggested that some of the "tiny bits" might be, at least partially, old habit. He had been in the depression whirlpool for so many years it makes sense that it could take some time to pull himself out of it.

When I asked each of them what their favorite part had been of their experience so far, I got three very different answers.
Quinn: "The intensity went away. I can breathe."
Dad: "I can talk to my son without fighting."
Mom: "Last week he said 'Mom, I think I really like myself.' That's a first ever!"

In asking them about the actual food on the Protocol, all three were rather blasé about it. "Oh, it's fine. It's not a problem." Evidently what many consider the most difficult or as some put it, the "impossible" part of the Protocol was very simple to them. Good! Of course, since this was 2009 there was now numerous excellent Paleo recipe sites, which have greatly facilitated the ability to comply with the dietary restrictions.

Since Quinn still had some underlying anxiety, not to mention some bad cognitive behavioral habits to break, they asked for a referral to a psychologist. I was glad that I was able to refer them to someone who is not only happy to work without medications, but who is actually familiar with my Protocol.

After all this happening in just thirty days, I was looking forward to seeing what would happen in the next month.

Follow-up:

Poof! I never saw or heard from them again. As I've said before, there are often one or more sensible reasons for this. Maybe it was the six-plus-hour drive, or maybe Quinn was just sick and tired of doctors' visits. Can't say I could blame the kid about that. Because Quinn could see and feel for himself what the Protocol had done for him, my thought is that he and his family stayed with it and they simply no longer needed me. Whatever the reason, again, it doesn't really matter. We had taken Quinn from suicidal to smiling, and that's the only part that does matter.

CASE STUDY 23

Height/Weight:

Blood type:

Blood pressure: "I'll be sober" husband/doctor

Comments: Rx: none   Fishoils

Notes:

Name: Allie V. (Female)

Age: 4
DX: None officially
Other diets: On GFCF

Again, although not officially diagnosed, I wanted to include Allie for many reasons. This definitely was a "worst case scenario" and yet it still worked. Her symptoms fit into both the Aspergers and ADHD categories, but I don't think I've ever seen such a prime example of ODD. I can't imagine what the parents' life was like with such a defiant, stormy child! This case is also an excellent example of the fact that even if the whole family is not on board, it still can be done. A dysfunctional family environment of course is not optimal, yet it can still be done. **But mostly I include this one because it graphically**

displays how the exact same trigger -- in this case the iron/manganese imbalance -- can cause different symptoms in many, or in this case all, of the family members. Allie was not as yet officially diagnosed, but her mom and dad both were.

Okay, I'm just going to say it. This one was a nightmare! I've had my share of tough kids and tough parents to work with, but this one was definitely in the top two or three in both of those categories. Maybe even number one...

Just to get things rolling, Allie was living in a violent and unstable household. Her dad was diagnosed as an "uncontrolled bi-polar" and he could very quickly and easily get violent. Her mom, a diagnosed schizophrenic, found my very simple paperwork "too hard" to fill out and left it blank. As it turned out it didn't matter. Allie's symptoms were very apparent.

Extremely hyperactive and nearly constantly screaming, she literally would not sit still for a second. In the course of our appointment her mom had to chase her down and bring her back several times despite my locking my office door. She even resorted to physically tackling her daughter at one point to prevent her from destroying my office. The worst and most chilling part of this is how much Allie enjoyed rattling her mom. The more upset she became, the harder Allie laughed and the more she pushed the envelope. When her mom would say "Allie! Sit down!" Allie would loom over her and repeat her words in a menacing sing song voice. I get along well with the majority of the kids I work with, and they will usually settle down, at least for a while, by my talking to them. When I tried to talk to her in my patented "firm disciplinary tone," which usually works, she narrowed her eyes at me like a cat, then very purposefully stood up and urinated all over herself and my office, laughing at the top of her lungs as she did so.

How do you deal with a child who has no reaction to discipline other than to enjoy it? Very articulate and verbally brutal, she had her mom in tears several times, then mocked her for crying. I can't accurately describe what this was like to watch! What could you possibly do with a four-year-old who acted like this, and more importantly, what would she be like by the time she was five? Or twenty? Holding a struggling and screaming Allie in her arms, her mom summed it up. "I can't take it anymore. I'm exhausted. We're all exhausted." I totally believed her. I had only been with her for 20 minutes and I was exhausted!

There have been a wide range of reactions I've seen over the years when I get into the specifics of the Protocol. They have ranged from "This is it? This is so easy!" to "This is impossible! You can't live without bread!" This was the first time anyone ever had such an extreme and unexpected reaction. As soon as Allie's mom started to go over the food list, she suddenly went into a full-blown panic attack! At first I thought maybe she was just being overly dramatic, but no, this was the real deal. It took quite awhile to get her calmed down, especially with Allie actively goading her. Despite all the people waiting for their appointments downstairs, my typical one-hour appointment was rapidly ticking into two.

When she had calmed down enough to speak, she kept repeating the same phrase. "I can't do this. It's too hard. My husband is going to freak out. I can't do this!" I let her go on for a while, simply because it didn't seem that I had any choice. When she ran out of steam I very calmly explained to her the Protocol was all I had to offer. There was no "magic pill," no "treatments" to do instead. I could give her guidance on the Protocol, but it was a take-it-or-leave-it situation. I told her that if she wanted to try it that she should start on Phase 1, and that she could get some recipes and advice about how to start from my staff. It's a good thing that my staff has gotten used to the uncomfortable situations in which I have had to sometimes place them, because they spent another two hours downstairs going over recipes with Allie and her mom. Bless their patience, because the only comment I heard from them was, "Is she alright?"

The next day:

It has long been my custom to take phone calls from 9:00 -10:00 am in my office. Sometimes it's just clients asking a quick question or for clarification, but over the years it has most often been strangers asking about the Protocol.

At precisely 9:00 am, Allie's mom was on the phone. She told me that her husband had indeed "freaked out" and wanted to make sure that there wasn't "just a pill or something" they could use instead. I again took over twenty minutes calming her down, all the while looking at the flashing red lights on my phone indicating all the calls I had stacked up. I explained to her that I needed to get to my other calls, but I had to all but hang up on her.

In the following days:

For the next two weeks, Allie's mom called every morning at pre-cisely 9:00 am. Eventually I told her that she couldn't take up my entire phone-work hour just for her every morning, as there were people calling from all over the world with their questions. When she did not stop, I explained to her that I would not be taking any more than two of her calls per week as she was monopolizing all the time available to others. Three of my staff also explained this to her when she continued to call every morning.

It didn't stop. When I stopped taking her daily calls, she started coming into the office and would proceed to bombard me with crying and questions when I came downstairs. All this drama unfolded unabashedly in front of clients who were sitting in the waiting room. She did this for several days until I took her aside and told her that

I would not see Allie anymore if she continued her behavior. She seemed to understand, and did indeed stop.

<u>One-month progress report:</u>

When I saw Allie's name on my daily appointment list, I steeled myself for another rodeo, and took everything off all the surfaces in my office. Especially anything sharp. When I went downstairs to greet them, I immediately noticed that they both looked better, more refreshed. A month prior, they both had very pronounced circles and bags under their eyes, especially Allie -- these were now gone.

Somehow, against extreme odds, her mom had managed to keep them both on the Protocol. This had to be nearly miraculous considering not only mom's emotional issues, but in one of the more cruel cases I've ever seen, her dad was taunting her with food not allowed on the Protocol. Just that morning he had been waving biscuits in Allie's face saying, "These are soooo good! Don't you want some? Here have some."

Allie was much, much calmer today, and the first thing she did was come around to my side of the desk, take my hand with both of hers, and apologize for "being such a brat" during the first appointment. In a bit of a daze, I accepted her apology. She gave me a smile and went to take her seat.

Mom was much calmer today as well, and said maybe she needed to apologize for being a brat too! She was staying on the Protocol with

Allie and was feeling less stressed and anxious as a result. It was decidedly odd to see them both sitting quietly in their chairs today. No screaming, no crying, no hysteria. What a relief! But it was also a powerful emotion that came from witnessing their improvement.

It hadn't taken long for the Protocol to show its first effects. Even while her mom was still making daily calls and visits to the office, Allie was already showing changes. "It was more me freaking out than her" admitted her mom. The hyperactivity was the first to go. It started to slow almost immediately and now at a four week mark was nearly gone. She was sleeping better, and her focus was improving. So much so that she had been voted "best behaved" by her teacher at school. "I never thought I'd see that day" said her mom with a heartfelt shake of her head.

The defiant and purposefully mean behavior that had been so alarming and prominent was virtually nonexistent. Her mom explained, "She can get triggered and be mean or yell if her dad has a bad episode, but she doesn't do it other than that." Poor kid. It wasn't hard to tell where she had learned that behavior from! "I was afraid she was bi-polar like her dad, but she's obviously not," she added. Allie smiled and touched her hand at that comment.

Another issue that I had not been aware of is that Allie had not been potty trained when we first saw each other, and that too had resolved itself in the last month. She had issues with constipation before that may have been holding her up, and eating the real whole foods and higher fats had resolved that problem. When the constipation stopped, so did her potty training problems. "She just did it herself from one day to the next."

Asking Allie to go downstairs to get her a drink of water, which she obediently did, her mom asked me some very specific questions about the Protocol and any possible effect on her husband's bi-polar issues. She herself was feeling so much better that she had a doctor's appointment to start weaning her off her prescriptions. I explained to her that I felt that the same high manganese that had caused Allie's problems, and possibly some of her own schizophrenia issues, could have some impact or effect in getting to the root of his bi-polar diagnosis. In any case, it couldn't hurt to try since it was just food. Sighing she said, "That's what you think." At the time I didn't really understand the comment, but I was about to be enlightened.

When we went downstairs, Allie was happily looking through our sticker collection we keep for the kids, and was discussing their various pros and cons of them with my receptionist. When she let out a girlish giggle at one of her comments, my receptionist, Rae, looked at me with the highest of raised eyebrows. I could read her mind -- "Is this the same kid?" We exchanged the same look a few minutes later when Allie spontaneously gave me a goodbye hug.

Follow-up:

Things apparently did not go well when the subject was broached that Allie's dad join the girls on the Protocol. Not only did he refuse the dietary change, he actually "forbade" Allie or her mom from ever seeing me again. Under the threat of violence, he had told his wife that he would "not allow her to spend so much money on Allie." She apologized profusely, thanked me, and told me that she would try to let me know how Allie was doing.

Despite this edict, she continued to try to keep up the very nominal supplements they were taking and somehow managed to stay on the Protocol. I didn't know this as she was just coming in and paying cash from time to time and I never saw her. My staff, of course, did not know that she wasn't "allowed" to be there by her husband. A few months later, we all got a wake-up call.

Coming down the stairs chatting with a client, I suddenly saw a man I had never seen before bolt out of a chair, point at me and yell,

"There you are!" He then unleashed the most vile, abusive, and pro-fane tirade I had ever heard. Most of it was just vulgarity (his cuss-word vocabulary was rather epic) and he also hurled insults such as "charlatan," "cheat," "snake oil," and "quack." It wasn't until he mentioned "Allie" that I had any inkling of who he was. What do you know? I was finally meeting Allie's dear old dad.

Just as he put his hands out in a "strangling" gesture and looked like he was going to come at me, and I braced for it, his eyes shifted to the stairs. Luckily for me at that moment, my six-foot tall brother, Doug, had just come down the stairs to see what the racket was all about. I guess Allie's paternal unit felt that he could handle little five-foot-four me, but Doug must have looked like too much chal-lenge. With a last burst of vulgarity, he abruptly ran out the door, to the relief of us all. My receptionist called 911 back with shaking fin-gers and canceled the call she had made during the loud and violent confrontation.

Again, against the odds, I did see Allie's mom again, just a few months ago. When I came down the stairs, she threw herself on me crying. Instead of the hysteria I had seen from her originally, this time it was gratitude. She started thanking me over and over again for giving her "such a model child" and wound up hugging not only me but my whole staff in her frenzy of joy. After talking with her about Allie's continuing progress for a few minutes, she wiped her eyes and took her leave.

It was at this point that, with a certain amount of embarrassment, I went over to greet the family that was waiting for me. As I started to apologize, the dad waved me off with a smile. Taking my hand in a handshake, he said, "Something tells me we're in the right place." This family was also there to see me about their autistic child and they took the gratitude they witnessed as a very good sign.

So why am I telling you this whole sad, strange story? **Because it proves once again that no matter what is coming against you, you can do this if you really want to!** Don't make excuses! It took an enormous amount of dedication and courage for Allie's mom to keep her on track. I witnessed first-hand for myself what kind of pressure she was living under. Maybe it isn't my place to think such a thing, but I fervently hope that she uses that courage to get both herself and Allie away from such a violent and abusive man. I will probably never know, but I can hope. All I know is that despite having the deck stacked against them from the start, Allie's mom committed to do everything she could for her child, and both she and Allie triumphed in the end.

CASE STUDY 24

Dad: *"Everything is one-hundred percent. Teachers are happy, we're happy, Avery is happy"*

Name: Avery W. (Male)

Age: 7
DX: ADD
Other diets: None. A lot of fast food and junk food. "We're really bad eaters."

A pivotal and powerful message I am trying to communicate through many of these case studies is that you can do this yourself! **This study more than proves it because Avery, a first grader, not only did this all by himself, he led his family to better health through his example.**

Many people are understandably skeptical about the Protocol. They worry about "excluding whole food groups," what they will eat throughout the day; many find it difficult to believe that what you eat can have such a dramatic effect on how you function. It goes beyond skepticism though when the very first words out of Avery's mother's mouth were, "I don't believe in diet or exercise." My response was to ask, "Then why are you here"? She turned away with a bored expression on her face. Luckily Dad was there to take over.

As it turns out the only reason they were here was because of an exceptionally strong recommendation from Avery's father's supervisor, whose son had also been through the Protocol. Because of their more casual work environment, Avery's dad had actually witnessed the process positively impact his supervisor's son, since the boy was frequently at the workplace.

You've heard it said that denial is a powerful master; denial was immediately and heavily apparent in this case. On the intake forms and in talking to the boy's parents, the only thing they were concerned about was his focus and grades in school. While I feel that grades are important, I was much more concerned about Avery's behavior. At seven, he was acting more like a fearful two-year-old. He whimpered and whined, and if he had a question he whispered it in his dad's ear to ask me. When I told him he could ask me questions himself, tears welled up in his eyes and he shook his head in a timid "no" gesture.

As I often do when I need a private word with the parents, I asked Avery to please go downstairs and get a file I needed from my receptionist. My whole staff knows that this is code for "try to keep him down there for awhile." Once he was out of earshot, I addressed my concerns about his behavior. As it turns out, it wasn't just me whom Avery seemed afraid of. He didn't talk to anyone except his parents, and only to his teachers when he had no other choice. Mom was rather affronted by this and asserted that he was "just shy," but the father intervened by telling her, "You know it's more than that." She shrugged.

Because I could hear Avery coming up the stairs, I quickly shifted gears back to his issues with school. His difficulties with school-work, particularly reading, began in pre-school. He had always had a hard time focusing and that lack was reflected in poor grades and a strong avoidance of doing any homework. His teacher at school said that if this did not change "very soon" she would have to recommend special ed classes.

During my discussion about the specifics of the foods allowed and not allowed on the diet, Mom actually got up and declared she was leaving several times. Every time I would make a recipe suggestion or tell them where they could get more, she would get disgusted. If I heard "this is so stupid" or "how ridiculous" one more time I doubt we would have made it through the appointment. Luckily again, Dad was still on board and was asking very specific questions about why certain foods were in or out.

After about a half hour of this, Dad too seemed to hit his limit. He expressed concerns that this would be "impossible" to do, and more specifically, that he didn't want to eat like this either! They were worried that Avery "would starve" without bread and I was told, "If he doesn't get what he wants he'll stop eating and starve." Since this was uttered in front of the child, basically giving him a guideline to follow to get whatever he wanted, I figured that the appointment was over. Then Avery, who I was not even certain was following what was going on, quietly voiced his opinion. Making eye contact with me for the first time, he asserted, "I want to try it." Turning to his dad, he repeated, "I want to try it." Sighing and settling back into his seat, his dad responded, "Okay, buddy," then asked me what they needed to do.

Buddy. First Mom proclaims to me, "I don't believe in diet and exercise" and now Dad is calling his son "buddy!" It was my turn to sigh.

Predictably, since his dad called him "buddy," there was a lot of "apologizing" for the rest of the appointment that he would have to "eat this terrible food." Terrible food? It was just *real* food! Mom asked specifically what drive-through food he could have. I said that there was currently no Protocol-compliant food available in drive-through (read "fast-food") places. "Sorry, buddy." Macaroni and cheese? "Sorry, buddy." Pizza? Aha! I had one! Digging some recipes for Protocol-compliant pizza I had printed out from a file folder, I handed them to his mom, who took a cursory look through them and pronounced them too difficult to make. She just wanted the frozen kind. "Sorry, buddy." In looking at his chart while writing this I noticed that I actually started counting how many times they said "Sorry, buddy." It came to fourteen by the end of the appointment. Not a good sign.

So here I had a first grader with two parents who were not going on the Protocol with him, and kept apologizing for making him eat real food. I couldn't help but feel that this one had a snowballs chance at best. Nevertheless, I gave Avery his own copy of the Protocol to take to school with him, and a pep talk about taking on responsibility for himself. I didn't say it out loud, but I knew poor little Avery was going to have to take this burden on his seven-year-old shoulders.

The predictable email:

"Avery has been on the spectrum diet for one week now. And I am totally frustrated. I don't know what to do to expand his menu! The only thing he will eat is a burger and sometimes chicken, clementines, carrots... We are talking breakfast and dinner. He refuses to eat lunch now. And he's starving all the time. I bought sweet potato chips for him, thinking it would be a snack food and he hates them. Same with sweet potato fries. I don't see how this much red meat can be good for him. He'd eat salad but he doesn't like oil and vinegar. I have no snacks I can pack for him for after school care. I've just about had it. I feel like he's being punished and so does he. You have

pumpkin on the list but I can't give him a spoon and tell him to go for it. I can't even make pumpkin bread as a dessert. I need some help with things I can make and real actual snacks. I don't know how we can keep this up for another month or two".

The only reason I posted this whole email is so that I could point out how mindset can sabotage this Protocol. Let's pick it apart...

1. On the diet for one week and she is "totally frustrated." I always tell people that change, especially major change, takes time. Somehow I don't think anyone would consider one week to be much time.

2. "The only thing he will eat..." Kids will eat when they get hungry, and they will eat whatever you give them. Avery's parents gave him a road map to get out of eating things he didn't feel like in the first appointment with the "starvation" thing. Can't blame the kid for trying to drive it!

3. "He's starving all the time." If he was truly starving, he'd eat. Get out of that mindset that if a kid skips a meal they're going to starve. True starvation is consuming very few calories for a prolonged period of time, leading to organ failure and death. This is a far cry from dealing with cravings as you wean off of atrocious "foods!"

4. "I bought sweet potato chips for him thinking they'd be a snack food. Same with sweet potato fries." This one is more subtle. Why does he need specific "snack" foods? Why not just snack on regular whole food, you know, like carrots? Chips and fries are not necessary for health. Looks like more of how she eats than him.

5. "I have no snacks to pack for him." Again the mentality that "snacks" can't be food, and that a snack only comes in a plastic wrapper.

6. "I feel that he is being punished and so does he." For the record, I never heard one word out of Avery saying that he felt punished. Granted he probably talks to his mother differently than he does with me but you'd think I'd get some inkling that he was unhappy. I think the more accurate statement would be that his mother was the one who was feeling "punished" because she had to figure out a new way to cook!

7. "I can't even make pumpkin bread as a dessert." I'm going to go ahead and put desserts in with "chips and fries." They are treats, not food groups, and are not supposed to be part of the Phase 1 Protocol anyway.

8. "I don't know how we can keep this up another month or two." This made me sigh as it showed her intention to go back to their sugar, bread, junk and fast food diet once Avery was feeling better.

As I said, this email was no surprise as I get them all the time. This was just a particularly good example of how people can self sabotage. For your edification, here is what I returned to her:

(My email): *"Sorry you're feeling this way, but there is not much I can say. Hundreds of people have been successfully through the Protocol without feeling that they are being "punished." The very fact that you say "I feel like he's being punished and so does he" is very telling. If your attitude is that he is being punished then he will feel the same way.*

"As far as expanding his menu, there are lots of different foods on the diet. Keep trying new ones until you hit on some he likes, or keep serving the same ones until his tastes expand a bit.

"Suggestions: We do have the recipes that I told you about available that some of our Spectrum moms have come up with. If you stop by we'll be happy to make you copies.

"When you came in you expressed a lot of doubt in spending this much time cooking and figuring out recipes. I understand that it is a challenge and a big change, but we have seen such great results using it that I would encourage you to continue. However, it will be your responsibility as the parent to come up with the food choices for each meal. We have provided all the guidelines, but you have to get it on the plate!

"Be Well: Shauna"

One-month progress report:

A month later, when I walked downstairs to greet them, a different boy was waiting. He popped up out of his chair with a wave, and came over to say hello. Grinning and easily making direct eye contact he informed me, "I'm going to want to ask some questions today. Is that okay?" I told him that is was not only okay, it was awesome! I got a big smile from that adjective.

His first question was regarding watermelon. He said it was on the "second" list, meaning in the moderate food category, but he was really missing it. So I asked him, "Can you be responsible about it, and not eat too much?" He looked over at his mom. Since I knew she was not being helpful about this, I drew the focus back to Avery.

Trying to take a light but deliberate tone, I appealed, "Don't look at her Avery, look at me. I'm talking to you and we're making a deal. Will you not eat more than two small slices at a time and not more than twice a week?" He joyfully agreed to my terms and we shook on it to seal the deal.

During Avery's first month on the Protocol, his focus had begun to sharpen almost immediately and his schoolwork was rapidly improving as a result. As his dad said with a smile, "The teachers are all saying thumbs up." Avery added to this by telling me, "My teacher says I'm reading circles around the other kids now!" He was very proud of his new successes and told me about all the glowing compliments he was receiving from his teachers. I let him ramble on because he had earned every one of those accolades, and I felt he deserved to toot his own horn for awhile. Especially since despite his success his parents were still not on the Protocol with him and his seven-year-old self was having to go it alone.

Since the schoolwork had been the parents' main concern in coming to see me, we discussed that first. Frankly I was more interested in the changes in Avery himself. Whiny and overly timid in his first appointment, he was now sitting excitedly on the edge of his chair, asking questions, talking about his challenges and successes, and participating fully in the conversation. He never stopped smiling the whole time, and his pride in what he was accomplishing for himself gleamed in his eyes. He was surprised to find that he felt much more relaxed and also how easily he was getting over his shyness around other people. Dad managed to get a word in edgewise here and agreed with his son. "Oh yeah," he enthused. "Avery actually went over to the neighbor's house and asked if he could use their basketball hoop. That's huge!"

At this point, I used excuse number two to get Avery out of the room by telling him he could go downstairs and find himself a sticker out of our collection. "Get the most awesome one, Avery, because you're so awesome," I yelled after him as he giggled and bolted noisily down the stairs.

Now it was tough time. I told the "adults" that I understood from Avery that they were not on the Protocol with him. Mom snorted, "No way. I'm not doing that!" Dad simply hung his head so I assumed that was a no. This was one of those times where it takes an effort of sheer will not to yell at people. Somehow, their seven-year-old boy could be responsible enough to completely change his diet and stick to it, but they, the so-called grown-ups, could not! Avery was even refusing food that his mom was giving him and would instead root around in the refrigerator for "something on his diet". She was sabotaging him and he was still standing strong.

Instead of the frustrated tirade I wanted to deliver, I decided instead to try to appeal to their common sense. "How can you not want to try this for yourselves? Since Avery has been on this Protocol you've witnessed with your own eyes how much change he's made." Dad's head was still hanging, but Mom gave me her answer -- "So?"

Two-month progress report:

There were big doings this month, and it wasn't all with Avery. Mostly for financial reasons, his parents had gone (mostly) on the diet with him. Mom was still eating some chips and sodas, but Dad had decided to go whole hog and see if anything would change with him. After only about two weeks, he was "blown away." I was thrilled that Avery was no longer alone.

This time It was Dad who was babbling. It seemed like he just couldn't say enough good things fast enough! Avery's school reports were all glowing. His focus was sharp and his reading skills were "going off the charts." His attitude was also being praised, as exhibited in one report shown to me: "Avery pays attention and he's the first one in his seat ready to go." When I asked the child how the homework avoidance thing was going, he shrugged casually and said, "Eh. No problem."

Next I asked him if it was easier now that the whole family was on the diet. He responded that it was, but quickly asserted that he had been handling it well on his own before they joined him. His dad emphatically confirmed, "He was amazing. He'd even refuse foods people tried to give him." Avery chimed in here because he wanted me to know that he had stuck to our watermelon agreement. "I'd only have two slices this thick, and no more than twice a week." This seemed to be a far cry from the infamous "he's being punished" email I had received, but I kept silent. Things were going great and I didn't want to toss a wrench in the works.

Three-month progress report: (Phone)

Since they live quite a distance away, I just got a phone call for the next check in. On my suggestion, Avery and his dad had read "The Paleo Solution" together and had decided that's what they were going to do "from now on." I will always bless Robb Wolf for writing a book that speaks so well to men!

When I asked if everything was still working, Dad enthused, "Everything is one-hundred percent. Teachers are happy, we're happy, Avery is happy." Good. Then I'm happy.

Follow up:

About six months after that last appointment I had with this family in 2011, I got a call from Avery's father. They were moving cross country and he wanted to say goodbye and to tell me how well Avery was doing. The kid was burning up the charts with his grades, and more importantly, he was happy. Truly happy. They were still very committed to staying Paleo and were getting into more of a groove of what to cook.

"I just had to call and thank you," Dad said. "Not only did you and this diet save our son, it saved the whole family." I reminded him that it really wasn't me. It was Avery! It's kind of a shame that the family had to be led by a seven-year-old, but I'm just grateful it happened. Who'd have thought it was even possible.

Whenever I've spoken with Avery, I always made it a point tell him how awesome he is. But he's more than awesome. He led his whole family into better health -- so in my book, he's more like a hero.

CASE STUDY 25

Mom: *"I've always known he was in there and now I'm seeing him. I promised him when he was little I'd come and get him, and now I have."*

```
Age: 11                                    VIT strength
DX: Autism = abnormality Chromosome 15
Notes:   No ages

Started SBP in March —
Wants to maximize benefits

Saw "amazing changes" first few
days = Wants it to continue
By 4th day was starting to have spontaneous
conversation
"We see flashes of brilliance"

Was on GAPS for 2 years = "I feel free —
this diet is so easy"
```

Name: Marcus P.

Age: 11 (turned 12 while I was working with him)
DX: Autism caused by **Abnormality Chromosome 15**
ND: Michael Kane
Other diets: GAPS for over 2 years, SBP for 1 month

Marcus is yet another child who I was never fortunate enough to meet in person. I would have loved to have witnessed this one with my own eyes, but it took place completely over the telephone. His case is extremely interesting to me not only because of the seemingly impossible results, but because this one case alone represents so many of the diverse situations I've seen in my dealings with hundreds of children. Even with both "modern science" and the "odds" stacked against him, Marcus, along with his very capable ND, and his dedicated parents, still triumphed.

In 2005 when I first started working with autistic spectrum disorders (ASDs), they generally were diagnosed based on the child's behavior. For example, ADD or ADHD were for the hyperactive ones. Aspergers was for the high-function kids who lack social skills. Autism was for those who were unaware of their surroundings, and PDD-NOS indicated that something is wrong, but had yet to be identified. I've always thought PDD-NOS was a singularly inconclusive "diagnosis."

By the time I first started working with Marcus I was seeing more and more people whose children had been diagnosed with some type of "genetic" autism. I am always careful about creating expectations for anyone trying the Protocol, yet it became even more dicey ground when I started seeing kids with diagnosed genetic modifications. I was very clear with them that I didn't know if it would work or not with a chromosome abnormality. Fortunately, it did for Marcus, and it has for others.

As I said, his situation was more diverse and therefore more difficult than most. First of all there was the genetic issue. Second, his symptoms were very severe, and third, he was nearly twelve. The Protocol generally works faster and more reliably on little kids, and Marcus was by now closer to the "young man" category. Setting realistic goals seemed important; it's just that as the years go on the idea of a "realistic goal" has become a moving target.

For the sake of brevity, I got most of this description of Abnormality Chromosome 15 from Wikipedia. Those people really know how to cut to the chase. In a nutshell:

"A specific chromosomal change called an isodicentric chromosome 15 (previously called an inverted duplication 15) can affect growth

*and development. In these situations, the affected person possesses
an "extra" or "marker" chromosome. This small extra chromosome
is made up of genetic material from chromosome 15 that has been
abnormally copied and attached end-to-end. In some cases, the extra
chromosome is very small and has no effect on a person's health. A
larger isodicentric chromosome 15 can result in weak muscle tone
(hypotonia), mental retardation, seizures, and behavioral problems. Signs and symptoms of autism have also been associated with
the presence of an isodicentric chromosome 15."*

So in other words, Marcus' autism was thought to be a side effect of
his extra chromosome. In addition to autism, he also had the weak
muscle tone, what appeared to be mental retardation, and behavioral
problems, so it all fit.

Diagnosed at age five, the family had tried multiple diets, supplements and therapies. Being on the GAPS diet for over two years had
helped enormously with his awareness and with his general physical
condition. Working with their talented ND had helped even more,
as Marcus was able to acquire some speech skills. Although he had
no spontaneous speech, he was doing something called "scripting."
If you've never seen this, it is quite remarkable. A child who has no
conversational skills at all will suddenly sing entire songs or recite
pages of dialogue from a movie without missing a word. No matter
how many times I see that, it is still uncanny.

On the advice of their ND, they decided to start Marcus on the Protocol at home on their own; we had not yet connected. For one thing,
they had no idea if it would be beneficial for them at all because of
the chromosome abnormality. His mom was thrilled when she saw it
because she felt it was much simpler than the GAPS diet he had been
on for over two years, so was more than willing to give it a whirl. It
was funny; I'm so used to people telling me that the Protocol is "too
hard," or "too much of a change." Imagine how happy I was when

some of his mom's first words to me were, "I feel free! This diet is so easy after being on GAPS!"

By the time I spoke to Marcus' mom for the first time, they had been on the Protocol for a mere few weeks. They decided to go whole hog on it and the entire family had embraced the change in diet in the hopes that it might help. They didn't have long to wait.

Almost immediately they saw "amazing changes" in him, she reported. On the fourth day on the Protocol, he started having spontaneous conversation for the very first time in his almost twelve years. After one week, while Mom was having a conversation and mentioned the TV show, "The Price Is Right," Marcus said, "Didn't Grandma always watch 'The Price Is Right?'" Yes she did. Since his grandma had passed away almost two years ago, his mom was thrilled to see that his memory was kicking in; something else he had never exhibited prior to now. After only a few weeks of dietary change, these results were rather stunning.

At only three weeks into the Protocol, his mom told me, "We are seeing flashes of brilliance." Committed completely to the Protocol now, she was taking very meticulous notes to make sure that she could prepare everything not just well, but perfectly. She asked many excellent questions, such as: if the food has to be all organic (preferable but no), if butter is okay (emphatic yes), and how to get more good fats into him (put butter, olive oil or coconut oil in everything!). I had a DVD I had created at the time explaining the Protocol, and she immediately ordered it. She was an absolute poster hero for how to do the Protocol and the results were already showing.

"Just tell me how to do this perfectly," she implored. "I want this to continue. It has to continue."

Part of the "amazing changes" that had already taken place before our first appointment was a lessening of virtually all the symptoms she felt needed to be addressed. Although he had started some spontaneous speech, it still had a very long way to go. The dramatic "melt-downs" that he had often been experiencing had ceased since he had started the Protocol, and they wanted it to stay that way!

Also notable since being on the Protocol Marcus had started following directions better, but there were "big gaps in his knowledge" of how to do things. His lack of fine motor skills had kept him from even being able to hold a pencil which was frustrating to him, but now he was showing interest.

When I asked at the end of the appointment if she felt ready, she laughed. "Let's do this thing!"

One-month progress report: (phone)

There was a theme to this appointment. I have never before or since had someone say, "I'm so grateful" so many times in the course of a half an hour.

The new changes were racking up so fast, she "didn't know where to begin," so I asked about their first concern; the lack of spontaneous conversation. That was changing and changing fast. He had started to be able to attend church "with the regular kids." Marcus was responding to questions, and constructing more sentences. Pretty advanced ones too! For example, he didn't just declare, "I love you", he expressed, "I love you because…" and would go on from there.

The "melt-downs" he had frequently been experiencing had simply disappeared. He had not had a single tantrum since starting the Protocol! This was evident when I asked his mom about them, as she said she had "almost forgotten" that he had ever had them at all. Even though they had experienced a severe tornado in their area this month, Marcus had remained calm.

Although there were definite gaps in what he knew how to do, Marcus was following directions much better and seemed desirous of doing what was asked of him. During a trip to the store, he surprised his mom by asking if they could buy some Lincoln Logs. Even though he had never played with toys in his life, she agreed, and both he and the family were having fun building with them.

At this point I suggested, as I usually do, that they try giving Marcus some chores that he was personally responsible for and could be proud of when he completed them. I also told her to be on the lookout for new changes. When your son suddenly starts maturing at such a rapid rate, it can be not only a shock to the system, but you can kind of forget that he is actually 12! You don't want to push him too hard, but it is often easy at this point to actually hold him back simply because you're not used to him being capable of so many new things. She promised that they would give that a lot of thought and attention.

Since they had been strictly adhering to Phase 1 of the Protocol, I suggested that she start introducing more Phase 2 vegetables and a little fruit and see if it made any difference. She was a little nervous about this, but it was the only way I could gauge where he was in his progress with the iron/manganese imbalance that was so obviously there. She agreed, but only if they could go back to Phase 1 if the progress stopped. I agreed fully with her there!

Two-month progress report: (phone)

As promised, the family had given a lot of thought to the notion that they might, out of love, be holding Marcus back a little. She admitted, "I know we're part of the problem. We do too much for him out of habit." They decided to start out by giving him more independence and Marcus was loving it. "He's much more spontaneous and social. He goes to church with a friend now instead of Mom and Dad. He's a super happy kid."

Instead of the cocoon of non-awareness that had previously shrouded Marcus' world, he was now "seeing the world around him." He was becoming interested in other people and what they were up to, watching TV programs with his family, and playing with new toys. He was getting interested in music and was performing "musical numbers" with his mom in the kitchen. Oh man, would I have loved to see that!

His conversational skills were becoming more complex and less self absorbed. He wanted to know what things were for, and was getting more interested in what they were eating. The move to Phase 2 of the diet had incurred no negative repercussions and he was having fun picking out what they would all have for dinner. "It's amazing. He'll actually tell you what he's thinking now."

Her ending comment "I can't wait to see what happens next" turned out to be prophetic.

Three-month progress report: (phone)

"I feel like we've really turned a corner here," Marcus' mom announced.

At the end of the previous week, Marcus suddenly made a "quantum leap" in sensory processing. Excited by the sudden progress, they decided to take him back to his ND to get him reevaluated. NDs use a sophisticated system of audio and visual processing to evaluate where in their learning curve a child currently falls. They assign numbers to these tests that correspond to the child's age; for example a five-year-old should be scoring fives on the tests, a ten-year-old should be scoring tens and so on. Marcus, who had just turned twelve, had been at a four on this scale prior to starting the Protocol. At this testing, he was at a nine, which is considered to be "the low edge of normal" for his age. Marcus had made five years' worth of progress in just over three months!

His conversations were becoming very exciting for his mom. He was having a lot more of them in general, and they seemed to be significantly more complex in both thought and speech. As a result he was becoming much more social and interested in other people. "He's inviting people into his world. That's not autistic," his mother declared.

With all of his other gains, his fine motor skills had also gone into high gear. Just in that month he learned how to tie his shoes, trace with a pencil, and was working twenty-four piece jigsaw puzzles by himself. His Lincoln Log architectural work continued to become more complex, while remaining just as much fun!

Now, equipped with a stronger base of knowledge and experience (as well as self-confidence and family support), Marcus was easily following instructions, and was not only doing his chores, but enjoying helping the rest of the family with theirs. "It's so cool! He's being diligent and meticulous," Mom gleefully noted.

With all the incredible improvements and changes in Marcus, this is often the time when many parents/families decide to rest on their laurels and become lackadaisical with the diet. Fortunately, that didn't happen in this case, because Marcus was not done dazzling us yet. Apparently, he wasn't about to let some pesky chromosome malformation get him down. No, Marcus was flying!

Four-month progress report: (phone)

With all of his leaps and bounds of progress, his mom and dad decided to try exposing him to even more new experiences to see how he would react. As his mom said, "It's time to open up his world now."

And open it they did -- wide open! They started taking him to movies, baseball games, all kinds of church and local events, even shopping malls. They took him out everywhere they could think of and he ate it up. "He loves them all. We take him places and then he discusses his experiences with us." The world was now open to Marcus, who was ready to see it all.

His motor skills were continuing to improve, and his jigsaw puzzles were getting larger and more complex. He now did all his chores around the house with no one having to prompt him or check that he'd done them correctly. "He's the closest to normal that he's ever been. I never thought we'd get this far."

When I asked about anything that still needed to be worked on, after some thought his mom replied, "Well, I wish I could get him to drink more water." We both had a good laugh about that one!

It was here, at the end of our four-month phone appointment that his mom said this to me. I know I opened the study with this quote, but I'm going to say it again because it is impossible for anyone to overestimate what it meant to me. As "professional" as I try to stay, it was a good thing I was on the phone at the time when she said it because I teared up. And I'm tearing up again just remembering it. Just before we said goodbye, she said: *"I've always known he was in there and now I'm seeing him. I promised him when he was little I'd come and get him, and now I have."*

When I hung up the phone, I reflected on what an honor that is. All those years that she would lay down on the bed with her non-responsive son and promise him that she was going to come for him. That she would bring him out into the world. And then... she did. Our world was now his world too. When I'm down, or tired, I think about how blessed I was to be able to help her keep that very important promise to her son. That's why I do this work.

Five-month progress report: (phone)

Since Marcus was continuing his rapid progress, we didn't even do our customary half hour monthly check in. I only spoke to his mother for about ten minutes this time. She just wanted to let me know that he was doing great. He was now bowling, enjoying baseball games and was learning to play catch.

I'm not entirely sure if this was a good thing or a bad thing, but he had also learned to sing, "Take Me Out To The Ballgame" (loudly) this month and was entertaining (??) them pretty regularly with this classic.

The family had traveled to go to a wedding this month, and Marcus once again stepped up to the plate. Spending all day at the wedding "shaking hands and speaking appropriately" had caused more than one relative to ask "Is that Marcus?" Yep. The *real* Marcus, who was once hiding in plain sight.

"What this diet has been all about is expanding his world," Mom described. "We never could do that before."

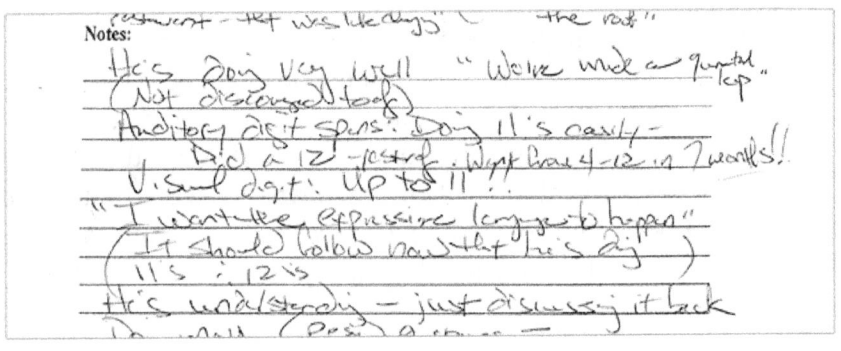

Six-month progress report: (phone)

At this six-month mark, Marcus had made yet another of his "quantum leaps." Suddenly his receptive language skills had "gone through the roof." So much so that they made another appointment with his ND for an evaluation. Although usually these tests only take place once a year, Michael was very happy to repeat his tests and gauge the new progress.

"It's getting ready to happen," Mom said with excitement. "The final chapter of his story is being written now."

She was right. **His processing skills, starting at four just six months ago, were now at an age-appropriate twelve.** With the odds definitely not in his favor to begin with, Marcus had made it.

When I asked if there were any issues left to work with, his mom said, "I'd like him to have a little more expressive language. But that's coming. We're not worried about that."

Follow up:

Shortly after our last conversation, a close family member of theirs passed away and communication kind of slipped. The last I heard from Marcus' ND, he said that the pre-teen was now being a pre-teen and doing great. I'm not worried about him. I'm sure that Marcus' story will continue to evolve.

It's enough to know that because of this Protocol, lots of people have been able to keep their promises to their kids. They kept the faith, they did the work, and sure enough, they went in and got their kids. I did my part, and that is after all, my job.

CHAPTER NINE

Raise The Bar!

Contrary to what you might think, the biggest stumbling block to this protocol has not been the kids not liking the food. As a matter of fact, after a brief adjustment period the kids usually love the food. It's the parents, and, sorry guys, but I have found through experience that it's usually Dad. Many dads just can't give up the fast food, chips, soda and bread. And mark my words, if those "contraband" items are in the house, the kids will find them and eat them. The general rule is if the kids don't see the items, they lose interest and desire for them very quickly. If they do see them, then you're probably in for some pretty serious and persuasive whining, or even a tantrum or two. And don't think that hiding spaces work -- curious kids will find them every time!

To be crystal clear: **90% adherence to this protocol will yield ZERO % result!**

That's why I always suggest that the whole family eat exactly the same foods, and that all "contraband" be removed from the house. Any time I have had a child that was making great progress who suddenly slowed or started to reverse, it has been because they found the "secret stash" that the parents believed was successfully hidden, sometimes even in a locked cabinet. Believe me, if there is even one "no-no" stash of snacks or soda or foods that don't belong in the house, your little cat burglar in training will find it, so do yourself a favor and ditch them.

It never ceases to astound me when I have heard the phrase "The Protocol is too much trouble" from parents. While I understand that change can be difficult, is a dietary change, even a significant one, really more troublesome than an autistic child? At first, I considered it just an excuse, and in some cases I still think it is, but over time my opinion has shifted.

Many of these families have nearly literally "tried everything". Diets, bio-medical interventions, ND's or other therapists, color/ light/sound therapies, ABA, essentials oils and swimming with dolphins. Most or even all of these have helped in some fashion but did not completely resolve the issues. Parents have become accustomed to settling for something that "helps," even if it's only a little. So when you confront such exhausted parents with the idea that they have to change their whole diet, their whole lifestyle in order to do this, some of them balk. It just seems like too much to do to create yet another of the slight changes they've experienced in the past, so they don't even want to try. **Although I can understand this mindset, you have to know that it is disastrous to the success you could achieve for your child using this Protocol.** *Please don't let that be you!*

And speaking of disastrous mindsets, there is yet another issue I never expected to encounter that is a rather new one. It's very odd to me but it's becoming so prevalent in the last few years that I feel like I need to address it. I touched on it briefly in the case study of Dylan D. but it bears repeating. Oh sigh… I wish I didn't have to because I'm just about to make a whole lot of people a whole lot of mad at what I'm about to say. I know this because of the amount of indignant emails I already get because I think that "autism needs to be cured". Ready? Here goes… There is a very large and very prevalent mindset beginning that the kids "are perfect the way they are". "It's not Autism - it's AWEtism"! Although I admire the idea that they love their children no matter what, I feel very strongly that this is not always in the best interest of the children themselves, and I feel that I must advocate for the children even if it upsets parents.

Hear me out. I have had more conversations than I could recount with the post-Protocol kids themselves who told me how unhappy they were feeling the way they did. Not only with the extreme sensory issues, nightmares, and not being able to express themselves, but with a more personal issue as well. *They want to grow up.* I often hear parents sigh and express the sentiment that "kids grow up so fast", and although this is a true and loving statement, it leaves an important part out of the equation. Kids are *supposed* to grow up. They want, *desperately* according to them, to grow up. So before you decide that your child is "perfect the way they are", please do one simple thing. Ask them. Ask them if they are happy the way they are. You may be surprised by the answer.

An unknown philosopher once said, "Doubt kills more dreams than failure ever will." I believe that with all my heart. It is so easy to doubt. Especially with something like this that literally seems too good to be true. If I've heard it once, I've heard it a thousand times: "If this diet is so great, why isn't everyone talking about it? Why aren't the autism societies embracing it? Why aren't you on 'Oprah' or 'Dr. Oz'"? That's legit. It does seem that with the increasing number of diverse cases showing the results I'm achieving, national appearances to discuss the Protocol would have followed.

One of the reasons certainly is because the families that have successfully been through it are mostly pretty quiet about it. If it were my kid I'd be yelling from the rooftops, but in reality, most just want to proceed on with their busy lives as if it never happened. You can't really blame them for that.

Another is that there are a ton lot of "autism specialists" out there and they all seem to have a different approach that they feel is best. If anyone else's approach falls outside their paradigm they have a tendency to dismiss it, sometimes without reading it or listening to success stories from their own patients. I, like them, feel I have the best approach (that's why we all do what we do) but I continue to do a lot of research and try to keep an open mind. My feeling is that combining different therapies is what will sometimes work best, but until you correct the iron/manganese imbalance? Well… in my opinion? I think you're swimming upstream. That's why so many therapies and diets seem to help for awhile, only to lose the ground again.

As far as to why I'm not being interviewed by respected TV show hosts? Hard to say. Maybe they are merely unfamiliar with my work, or maybe the pharmaceutical and breakfast cereal sponsors of their shows gave it the thumbs down. Quite frankly, the only reason I would even seek anything like that is to further spread the word that there IS hope for families who have autistic children, which is why I wrote this book. So in reality… mission accomplished. I now have you to spread the word.

Autism is not only crippling children, it cripples entire families. Some examples I've seen are a mother who no longer has an ability to work if she wants to, as her child can't attend regular schools or daycare and has to be constantly minded. Other children in the family can't go to preferred schools or do fun after-school activities because there is no money left to be spent on them, and the idea of a family vacation is a foregone conclusion as the affected child would never be able to behave and/or cope. A father who has to stay in a job he hates because he can't afford to lose his insurance. Families who can't live where they want to because they need to be in a system that caters to special needs children. The divorce rate is staggering, with some statistics showing over eighty percent of marriages with special needs kids ending in divorce.

With so many children affected, who will be our future leaders? Our poets? Our scientists? Autism is not only ruining the intellectual future of our country, it will ultimately contribute heavily to its financial and economic collapse as the insurance industry will be further pressured into absorbing the exorbitant medical costs associated with it. Costs that no country would be equipped to absorb.

The only real answer to autism is not treatment - it is eradication! Only by eliminating it will the tremendous physical, emotional, and financial drain end.

Am I saying that my dietary therapy will work with all autism, all ADD/ADHD, all ASDs? Of course not. *However, what I am saying that it has proven to be extremely effective when a component of a person's problem may be excess manganese.* Just think about it; if we could get rid of the majority of these cases by simply changing their diets, think of how the funding that is available could be so much better utilized for the cases that aren't manganese-related.

What I will tell you is that the food protocol, often used all by itself without any supplementation, has produced everything from mixed positive results to full reversals and re-diagnosis. This eliminates the need for expensive and invasive medical testing to see if their manganese is high, because the remedy is just food! And as I've said, the tests are not always even a good indicator. Most tests will only show what amount is present, and it is the *sensitivity* to manganese that is the culprit. Just change their diet for a few months. That will give you all the information you need to know.

The standard Paleo/Primal diet has practically become mainstream at this point, as so many have adopted it for the huge rewards in health and well being that they experience as a result. Did you know that "Paleo" was the number one most searched term on Google for 2014? Because of this, there are a literal plethora of recipe and lifestyle websites, books and blogs that can assist you in this new way of eating, and help you to make it fun and easier. **Although the Spectrum Balance® Protocol is considered to be a Paleo diet**

(since it eliminates phytates) it is still a very important targeted tweak away from a standard Paleo diet. By specifically addressing the iron/manganese imbalance that tweak can make all the difference in the world. So use the Paleo recipe sites, but be very mindful of the "avoid" food list of the Protocol.

This is an easy, healthy, non-toxic and no-harm way to try to create lasting and remarkable change. Even in the absolute worst-case scenario where the child doesn't radically change, the only downside is they ate healthier for a few months. Not much of a downside as downsides go. Give it a try for at least ninety days and see what happens.

Over time I have come to realize that the greatest obstacle to people trying this Protocol is that they have a very low bar of success. After years of "trying everything," they start thinking in very limited terms about what they want for and from their children. Many parents are no longer even daring to think in terms of their children graduating from school, getting a job they love, getting married and having kids themselves, or any of the many things parents dream about for their kids. Instead they are merely hoping that their children will become a little more verbal, to be able to feed themselves, or become less violent.

So let's go to work on re-setting that bar! Think about it for a minute. What do you really want for your little Janie or Johnny? Not what you've gotten used to wanting, but what you pictured in your head when you first knew you were going to have a baby! Go ahead, close your eyes right now and really picture it. Is it your son in his cap and gown celebrating with his friends? Maybe your daughter walking down the aisle? Your child's name in gold letters on the CEO's door? Publishing their first novel? How about the first time you hold your brand new grandchild? Now with those images in your head, with *your newly set bar*, does a change in diet really sound so difficult?

The current paradigm of autism and other related disorders is, "There is no known cause, no known treatment, and no known cure" or, in other words, there is no hope. Don't buy into that. *Right this minute, you are holding hope, right here in your hands...*

The Spectrum Balance® Protocol is backed by decades of nutritional and scientific research, but the kicker for me is that I've *watched* it work. Me, myself, with my own eyes. It has a track record of nearly a decade of dramatic and quantifiable *results*. And as you've probably figured out by now, I have kind of a pattern. I'm all about the results.

Be Well...

CHAPTER TEN

THE
SPECTRUM BALANCE® PROTOCOL

At long last, here we are at the end. The answer to the question you've been asking since the beginning of this journey. What are we going to eat?

Included here is not only the diet, but the whole document that has been downloaded ten's of thousands of times, and in over 67 countries. It will repeat most of the information that was covered in this book, but I want you to see what we have been offering *free of charge* for nearly ten years. As I stated before, I am writing and speaking right now and not seeing clients. We can still offer support through the NoHarm Foundation.

Although we encourage donations, it is important to understand that even with the publishing of this book, it will remain a free download available through the NoHarm Foundation.

Autism Paradigm Shift
An International Public & Professional Release

The Urgent Need to Embrace Nonconforming Thought
And a Return to Nutrition and the Natural Medical Sciences
In Effectively Conquering Current and Future Occurrences of
Autism Spectrum Disorders and Many Related Conditions

Presented by
No Harm FOUNDATION, INC.
NATURAL OPTIONS FOR HEALING AND RECLAIMING MEDICINE
A Colorado Not-for-Profit Organization
150 Rock Point Drive, Suite C Durango, CO 81301
Phone (970) 403-0817 Fax (970) 385-5834
www.noharmfoundation.org info@noharmfoundation.org

And

Assertive Wellness®
Research Center
Shauna K. Young, PhD, CTN
150 Rock Point Drive, Suite C Durango, CO 81301
Phone (970) 385-7577 Fax (970) 385-5834
www.assertivewellness.com drsky@assertivewellness.com

Copyright 2008-2014: Assertive Wellness Center, Inc. & No Harm Foundation, Inc.

Keynotes of this Revision for Our Current Users

Over the last several years, our commitment and promise to all of you has been to continue to use all resources available to us to provide through this website our best and updated dietary recommendations for our program. After much thought regarding nearly another full year of clinical experience combined with more and more reports back from participating families all across the country and beyond, Dr. Shauna has made the confident decision to cut all grains completely out of the Spectrum Balance® Protocol (SBP) - even within the Phase 3 long term lifestyle guidelines. This represents the most noticeable and important changes for this revision of the diets and the accompanying documentation.

To be truthful, the only reason that some grains were included in SBP in the very beginning and have not been totally eliminated prior to now is because so many people have felt that they could not even "attempt" the diet without at least some cereals, rice and/or pasta being included, since grain-based foods often represent the bulk of what children are accustomed to eating prior to starting the Protocol. So with reluctance we have tried our very best to permit only moderate amounts of the least objectionable suspects. However, time and ongoing research has shown us that grains of any kind (gluten-containing or not), even in extremely limited portions, will slow the positive process in virtually every case, and will stall out completely or reverse progress in others. So now we must adopt the very strong recommendation that you eliminate them completely from the diet **for the entire family**.

We discussed within our last revision that the Spectrum Balance® Protocol has most in common with a "Paleo" dietary philosophy, in that we eliminate grains and legumes and greatly restrict dairy. Many have expressed the notion that they are "looking forward to going back to their old eating habits", so let's dispel that right here. Although there will most likely be a time after you've achieved the positive results you're looking for that you can loosen the SBP dietary restrictions and follow a more generic Paleo-style diet for maintenance, there will **never** be a time when we will advise you to return to eating grains, legumes, sugars and processed foods loaded with additives if you expect and desire to maintain your health.

This Protocol was originally created to try to produce a positive response in symptomatic children, along with the hope that they will not always be as sensitive to the "no-no" foods. But this doesn't diminish the fact that some foods will just never be good for them - or good for the rest of the family either for that matter. Although we feel that wheat represents the most problematic grain and soy the most problematic legume, all of the members of these two food groups produce various degrees of negative effects, so you must do your very best to concentrate on the many forms of superior nutrition available to you. The human body is just not designed to process or efficiently utilize seed-based foods and they will never do anything but clog up your system and make you prone to disorders and disease of all types.

We continue to find that if you have a variety of creative recipes on hand, it really eases the transition to avoiding these problem foods that most of us seem to like and crave. Currently, one of the best recipe resources can now be found in the growing abundance of Paleo recipe websites. Many of these recipes can be used with SBP without any variations, and others can be easily modified by just omitting or substituting for "forbidden" ingredients like nuts during Phases 1 & 2 only. For example, we recently Googled "Paleo sweet potato recipes" and got 290,000 results. "Paleo rice recipes" got 577,000 and Paleo pasta recipes got 470,000. So give it a solid try because it will all be worth it to your family's precious health.

Our Ongoing Work

The No Harm Foundation was formed in 2008 with the core mission of providing a global conduit for badly needed information, education and support for the public and medical practitioners of all types regarding the proven connections between improper nutrition and the perplexing worldwide explosion in Autism Spectrum Disorders (ASD's), as has been pioneered through the research and clinical work of Dr. Shauna Young and her Assertive Wellness Research Center of Durango, Colorado.

Since that point in time it has become exponentially apparent to us that improper and inadequate early nutrition not only represents the primary etiology for the vast majority of occurrences of ASD's, but also both the causes and root answers for virtually all of the major maladies that are negatively affecting the fetal, infant and child populations of this planet. All the new drugs that will ever be created in attempts to prevent and cure disease will pale in comparison to the incomparable power that our bodies obtain from proper and natural nutrition, and much more of the world needs to rapidly acknowledge, embrace and broadly implement such intelligent and cost-effective strategies.

Effective modern nutritional and natural medical science is not currently seeing anywhere near their positive global implementation potential, yet effective, affordable and actionable answers for dramatic reductions in virtually all of these negative conditions that are impacting our youth as well as adults are already developed and presently available. Quality whole foods and countless natural medicinal remedies are capable of delivering health answers at fractions of the expense and hazards associated with pharmaceuticals. The public just needs to become aware of this.

The most recent statistics reveal that the destructive disorder of Autism now impacts in the U.S. alone, an unconscionable 1 in 60 children. Putting this figure in tragic perspective; that's more kids than are being stricken by diabetes, AIDS, cancer, cerebral palsy, cystic fibrosis, muscular dystrophy and Down Syndrome – **all combined**. After the hundreds of millions of public, corporate and governmental dollars that have been thrown at this one problem alone to date, the only real result we're all seeing is progressively worsening numbers. The social and financial implications for our world from this and other avoidable medical abominations are both staggering and expanding, and yet we see this dark and looming forecast as greatly avoidable.

We at the No Harm Foundation have been working diligently on behalf of the countless millions of affected families out there who need real, actionable and affordable answers for the health of their families – not a generation from now, not ten years from now…but *now*. In the midst of this highly challenging worldwide economy and exacerbated healthcare crisis, very few of these families possess the hundreds if not thousands of dollars a month that are required under many current drug and other therapy models in inadequate management of such destructive conditions as Autism. Although the various political factions may disagree as to how to make the system work best, all can agree that we need to save on costs so that available resources can be better reserved for those most in need.

Our capabilities are to *prevent* countless new cases of adverse medical disorders and to offer families already affected new treatment options – low-cost, non-invasive, non-toxic and effective options that virtually anyone can afford to implement, and without risk. We believe that these same discoveries may also be destined to bring positive redirection and new hope for many predominantly adult mental disorders such as *OCD, Chronic Depression, Bipolar/ Schizophrenia and Alzheimer's*.

In the face of disturbing international statistics for infant mortality, malnutrition, growth disorders, child obesity and learning &

behavioral disorders that include ASD's, which are all rapidly collid-
ing with diminishing private and governmental economic resources
to attempt to adequately address and mitigate such problems, it is becoming obvious that the only methods that will reverse the disturbing
trends involve delivering modernized education along with superior
and sustainable sources of foods and other nutrition as opposed to
relying on preventative and treatment strategies that will necessarily involve pharmaceuticals and other costly and even potentially
dangerous healthcare practices. It is painfully clear that the current
paradigm is no longer working in broad application.

It has certainly been our hope and expectation that by freely
releasing the vast majority of Dr. Young's building research and
clinical data into the public domain, we would see an exponential
bloom of collaborative participation by countless other researchers
and practitioners around the globe that would assist us in advancing,
perfecting and implementing what we have proven to ourselves and
countless others in order to accelerate positive change on a worldwide basis. Yet it has become obvious to us, especially over the last
couple of years, that our highly anticipated *passing of the baton* with
best intentions that we orchestrated, will not alone be sufficient to
stimulate in adequate time the paradigm shift that we see as absolutely necessary to take global nutrition practices and health management
along the paths that will start reversing the statistics in disease and
disorder back in the right direction. So the mission goes on.

Our paradigm-breaking work that has demonstrated the linkage
between nutritional imbalances and deficiencies with Autism Spectrum Disorders as well as a broad assortment of other disorders that
are impacting the youth and adults of our world, represents the first
and best hope in making true and sustainable change while there's
still time to reverse the alarming negative trends in avoidable disease
and death, and mitigate the unaffordable associated financial stress to
government at all levels.

We intend to network and partner with numerous individuals, companies, agencies and other humanitarian organizations worldwide to research and develop technologies, combine resources and facilitate projects that will fill in parts of this crucial global endeavor, and to take a leading role in bringing viable, affordable, actionable and sustainable sources of nutrition and natural medicinal resources to the peoples of our world. We always look forward to discussing any forms of sponsorship, partnering, media exposure or other promotion and support that will serve to advance these crucial goals.

NO HARM FOUNDATION, INC.
NATURAL OPTIONS FOR HEALING AND RECLAIMING MEDICINE

SUPPORT OUR GLOBAL MISSION

PLEASE HELP US PROMOTE REAL AND PROVEN SOLUTIONS FOR CHILDREN AND ADULTS SUFFERING WITH AUTISM, ADD, ADHD AND OTHER AUTISM SPECTRUM DISORDERS

Since 2001, I have had the pleasure of serving as General Manager of the Assertive Wellness Research Center located in Durango, Colorado, and over that time I have been witness to nearly miraculous reversals in the health and wellness of a great number of individuals with highly-varied ailments and conditions who have had the confidence to travel to the Center from every U.S. state and a number of foreign countries, solely as the result of private and professional referrals.

One of the most astounding testaments to the power of natural medicine and proper nutrition that we have experienced has centered around my sister Dr. Shauna Young's work for more than four years now with a multitude of children and adults who had been suffering under the symptoms that have been clinically diagnosed as **Autism, Attention Deficit Disorder (ADD), Attention Deficit Hyperactive Disorder (ADHD), Asperger Syndrome** and other closely-related learning and behavioral conditions cast under the ever widening net of **Autism Spectrum Disorders (ASD's).**

Through her intuition, clinical experience and persistence, Shauna has rediscovered a long ago identified condition of toxicity and imbalance in the human body that appears to demonstrate a direct link in causation to a good percentage of cases of ASD's, but even more important, she has also theorized and subsequently clinically-proven time and time again that a safe, uncomplicated and inexpensive dietary and supplement protocol is capable of producing rapid, undeniable and apparently non-regressing reversal and/or elimination of symptoms in an unbelievably-high majority of the cases that she has worked with.

So right up front, here are the bullet points on what you're probably looking for:

• Shauna's work has proven to us that not only is there a common link to many cases and syndromes along the Autism Spectrum, but that in a large percentage of such cases we find that the conditions and symptoms are *highly and rapidly reversible*

• Such effective reversals of symptoms can in many cases be achieved with no more than implementation of uncomplicated and manageable changes in diet, and the first noticeable incremental improvements can usually be measured in days and weeks as opposed to having to wait many months and even years

The primary goal of the No Harm Foundation is to aggressively help in getting this highly important message out to the general public and media with the hope that countless other medical practitioners will be stimulated and encouraged to join Shauna in making this information and help available to their clients and patients, and that the research and application of this productive new direction of medicine will be magnified a thousand fold worldwide.

This is highly-important subject matter and we truly hope that this material will start to supply part of the answers that you and countless other families are searching for. Please understand that this story has been a very difficult and a regrettably-long process in getting out, and although certainly not all of your questions will be answered in this writing, it is our most sincere goal that the broad public release of this information will spark and usher in an entirely new paradigm in research and real help for countless suffering children and adults.

Our extreme preference with this writing would have been to be able to supply you with a list of trained practitioners local to you, but regrettably that resource does not yet exist. There is no doubt that the potential for maximum individual success increases greatly where one-on one assessment and consultation with a healthcare professional is possible. However, due to the fact that enough of Shauna's clients have shared no more than their copies of her dietary protocol with friends and relatives who have reported being able to achieve various levels of undeniable success on their own, we have reached the point of confidence that a good deal of benefit can be achieved at home until greater resources become available.

We know that surely some percentage of those who decide to follow this Protocol will achieve no dramatically apparent result without individual professional assistance, but the potential upside here definitely justifies giving it a try. There's certainly nothing to lose, and everything potentially to gain.

As there is no way that Dr. Shauna's office is able to personally and effectively answer all your questions by phone, email or otherwise, we hope that the information you will find here will be able to address many of the issues and questions that she regularly hears from all around the country and beyond. After reading this information completely, we will do our best to help you where possible with your remaining questions if you will email to info@noharmfoundation.org or phone the Assertive Wellness Research Center in Colorado at (970) 385-7577.

If you are a physician, therapist or other healthcare practitioner and would like more information about participating in this program, you may also call (970) 385-7577 Tuesday through Friday (Mountain Time). Be sure to register your email with us through our website at www.noharmfoundation.org so that we will be able to keep you posted on new developments, protocol revisions, and on upcoming seminar and training resources that will be organized at the earliest opportunity.

We sincerely hope that you elect to join and help us in this worthy & necessary effort

DISCLOSURE & DISCLAIMER

The entire contents and information provided in this writing are intended only as a free-sharing of knowledge resulting from private research and clinical experience, and represents only the opinions of Shauna K. Young, PhD, CTN of the Assertive Wellness Center, Inc. Neither in her capacities as a practicing Traditional Naturopath nor as a Doctor of Philosophy in Natural Sciences, does Dr. Young diagnose or treat any disease or give out what is legally-deemed, "medical advice".

It is important to understand that the Spectrum Balance® Protocol & Diet have been created to address the theorized condition of abnormal and unmanageable stress being induced on the body, and the brain specifically, due to specific chemical disruptions associated with mineral imbalances that may result from improper nutritional choices. It is proposed by Dr. Young that by effectively restoring these balances with specific corrective dietary changes, many subjects may experience and have experienced reductions and/or elimination of some or all of the symptoms that have been classified under clinical labels such as PDD-NOS, Attention Deficit Disorder (ADD), Attention Deficit Hyperactive Disorder (ADHD) and various degrees of classic Autism. As these syndromes and disorders have not been formally classified by any medical body or authority as "diseases", then successful instances of reduction and/or full reversals of symptoms should not be in any way referred to as "cures".

No official clinical trials and/or double-blind tests have been conducted using this Protocol and it has not been endorsed by the U.S. FDA or any medical body, agency or association. This entirely new field of study warrants significant additional research and much broader clinical application, and the authors make no representations whatsoever that following this Protocol will provide the same level of desired progress for all subjects, especially when considering all the various underlying and unknown factors that may be present in each individual case and without each subject having the ability to receive personal consultation and assessment with Dr. Young or another trained healthcare professional.

This writing was not created and is not presented to be a technical paper and it was prepared most importantly so that the material could be easily understood for education of and consideration by the general public. The information contained is only provided for educational purposes and is not intended to replace a one-on-one relationship with a qualified healthcare professional. Dr. Young encourages each and every one of you to always make your own health care decisions based upon your own desires and research, and through consultation with trained practitioners.

Dr. Young is herewith making no philosophical, cultural, religious, environmental or other such judgments about the foods recommended or discouraged, and certainly you will need to take into account any foods that you or your children have known allergies or other sensitivities to. The Spectrum Balance® Dietary Protocol is not derivative of any other dietary philosophy to Dr. Young's knowledge and is definitely not consistent with all requirements of classic gluten-free and/or casein free (GF/CF) dietary protocols. Therefore, any child or other person who has received evidence by testing of sensitivities/allergies to these or other dietary factors should exercise proper caution with deviation from any special diet that is currently producing positive and cumulative results.

These statements have not been evaluated by the U.S. Food and Drug Administration. No protocols, foods or products herein discussed are intended to diagnose, treat, cure or prevent any disease, or to replace the need for regular medical care. If you are pregnant, nursing, taking prescription medication or have any medical condition, consult with your physician before making significant changes in your diet and/or supplementation.

THE SPECTRUM BALANCE® DIETARY PROTOCOL OVERVIEW

Shauna K. Young, PhD, CTN

I first theorized and began creating and making test use of the initial version of this dietary therapy in June of 2005, which I referred to at that time as the "Popeye Protocol". Since then I have continued to lecture, give seminars and refine the Popeye Protocol through my clinical work. The most recent version of this work that you now have in your possession is now entitled the "Spectrum Balance® Protocol", or as often referred to later in this writing as the "Protocol" or "The SBP."

This represents a very manageable, risk-free and inexpensive option that has resulted in the spectacular results we have seen with the many children and adults we've worked with for more than five years now. Although the period of time needed to achieve results has varied depending on individual factors and especially with regard to how well the subjects (and/or their parents) have followed the dietary guidelines, the usual response time for the first significant changes to be noticed have been averaging between 10 and 30 days. Think about it - worst case, the child does not respond, but still suffers no side-effects resulting from eating a healthier-than-normal diet for a few weeks. Best case scenario, a completely noticeable and improved situation by the end of a few months, and at extremely minimal cost and complication. This simple and inexpensive Protocol, time after time has resulted in complete & sustained reversals of symptoms regardless of the person's age.

Believe it or not, I have been talking about this program and my findings to whoever will listen in the global medical communities *for nearly ten years now*. I also began speaking with a number of the prominent Autism groups and found that nearly all of them declined to even go as far as to watch a video recap on DVD of several of my formerly Autistic, ADD and ADHD kids and their Mom's telling their own stories. There are absolutely no rational and logical reasons for this.

I finally came to realize that part of the problem is that the sheer simplicity of the Protocol makes it difficult to accept the results we're regularly seeing. It's extremely difficult to believe that something as simple as avoiding certain foods and adding other foods, some fatty acids and many times a few common supplements to a person's diet could have such profound impact, but as a Naturopath I understand that life often hands us these simple and natural solutions. So instead of continuing to lecture to skeptical organizations and more clinical ears, I reached the decision to start bringing my work directly to the people who seem most willing to listen and believe – **the parents**.

The clinical diagnosis of Autism is often considered to be a permanent brand not only on a child, but on the entire family: One that causes medical science to stop looking for any kind of cure and instead merely to cast around for something that might *help*. With most recent estimates showing 1 out of every 60 children (and growing) now being diagnosed Autistic, and many more somewhere else along the Autism Spectrum (ADD, ADHD, PDD, Sensory Integration Disorder, etc.), something obviously needs to be done to stop this horrible progression.

We have no doubts that there are numerous contributing factors to the development of Autism and other ASD's. I am constantly asked about the vaccine damage controversy. Although many parents have reported by their own observation, rapid onset of symptoms in their children closely following vaccinations, it is obvious that the majority of children who are vaccinated continue to be asymptomatic with regard to ASD's.

Let me just say right here that while I'm definitely no fan of vaccines, I do always support whatever informed choices parents make for their own children. Although I do not feel that vaccine damage is by any means a lone cause of the problems, I like many practitioners and researchers believe that they may act for some children as "the last straw" so to speak in cascading into these syndromes. It is very questionable as to whether this will ever be specifically proven (and admitted to), so we hope that vaccination will always remain a choice and decision for each informed family to reach independently.

How about genetic links? With as much energy and research as is being put into addressing this question, I have seen no data that evidences any more than minuscule genetic commonality for the disorders. Might there be some level of genetic predisposition that makes one child more prone to developing these conditions than the next? Sure; but where the allopathic medical community seems always obsessed with labels and categorization for every state of disease and disorder, the job of a good Naturopath is to be less concerned about specific causation of symptoms that have been clumped under a label, than to just look for what's necessary to try to reduce and eliminate them.

So what do I personally and professionally suspect is the primary culprit in causing these devastating symptoms? Although without question there are many possible contributing and complicating factors, I believe that potentially a very large number of these cases may be brought on and/or exacerbated by no more than an intolerable excess of the mineral/metal **manganese** in the brain that has accumulated due to over-consumption and other exposure, combined with insufficient bio-available iron and simultaneous suppression of the normal and natural regulatory mechanisms that our bodies use to naturally keep such an imbalance from occurring.

We refer to this imbalance as **"Menefe Syndrome"**: "Mn" is the periodic symbol for manganese and "Fe", the symbol for iron. Mn &

Fe sounded out together equals "Menefe". I know that many doctors and researchers often take pride in naming syndromes and diseases after themselves, but I never cared too much for labeling a condition that attacks millions of children worldwide the "Young Syndrome", or the like. So Menefe it is...

A little general info about manganese is warranted here. Manganese is one of those trace nutrients one wouldn't normally consider giving a lot of thought to, as our bodies usually maintain its levels in regular fashion. It is a naturally-occurring mineral that is found in many types of rock. Sometimes referred to as the "brain mineral", small quantities are important in the utilization of mental capacities and functions as well as in the formation of tendons, ligaments and in maintaining the structural integrity of the lining of various organs. But obviously the "brain mineral" idea caught my attention.

The first medical record of suspected problems associated with environmental overexposure to manganese was noted in 19th Century miners and was commonly referred to by the syndrome originally labeled "Manganese Madness". This was more-accurately cases of manganese "toxicity" as compared to what we are classifying as the Menefe Syndrome, however it was very instructive to find that the sufferers of Manganese Madness were nearly always in a state of **high to extreme sensory overload**.

This condition that afflicted these manganese miners exposed to toxic dust, appeared to cause symptoms of "emotional liability, irrationality, hallucinations and impulsivity". Chronic exposure led to "muscular weakness, ataxia, tremors, immobile facial expressions and extreme speech disturbances". These symptoms, often mistaken for Parkinson's in adults, also sounded to me suspiciously similar to Autism in a child. Further reading revealed that other very common symptoms of manganese excess can be speech difficulties and extreme reactions to sensory input - light, touch, smell and sound.

The neurological aspects from this overload are most likely due to the fact that the primary site of internal collection for manganese (described in neurological textbooks as "a neurotoxic metal"), regardless of the source of exposure, is the basal ganglia; the mass of nervous tissue buried within the cerebral hemispheres of the brain that is closely associated with the other nerve cell collections of the thalamus and hypothalamus. Since this nerve collection center is primarily responsible for coordinating and smoothing out the movements of the body and for organizing the sensory messages being sent to the cerebral cortex, it's no wonder that the neurological symptoms can the first to appear.

Abundant international research studies have been completed over decades that well-document not only the consequences of manganese overload in compromising brain function in animals and humans, but that adequately describe this competitive game of musical chairs so to speak that is competitively played between manganese and iron in a crucial brain chemistry balancing act. Again, the point of this abbreviated writing is not to overcomplicate this science for the reader, but anyone who wishes to perform a basic Internet search will locate an abundance of documentation on this subject.

Illustrated very simply, try to picture the consequences of this sensory overload in this way: Three people are in a room together trying to listen to me explain this concept. Unfortunately there are ten television sets that are all on different channels blaring away at top volume. There are also ten radios blasting away on ten different music stations. How will these subjects react?

• Let's say that Person #1 keeps darting from input source to input source; their attention being caught by a word or phrase coming from one of the TV's or radios only to be distracted again by something else being said on another station, and so on. This very quickly becomes exasperating

• Person #2 thinks to them-self, "Forget all this noise! I'm going to concentrate on this one TV screen and see if I can figure out what's going on". They concentrate and concentrate – even going so far as to repeat the words and phrases being heard in an attempt to be able to retain any information to the exclusion of all the noise going on around them. They may even strike out, rave or shout if someone disturbs them in their concentration

• Person #3 just can't handle all the input! They put their hands over their ears, close their eyes and shut down. If you try to penetrate in, they strike out to protect their fragile peace from the intolerable noise and input

According to medical science, Person #1 might be considered to have ADD, Person #2 – Asperger Syndrome, and Person #3 - Autism. All of these conditions manifesting differently in various people, but in response to identical input. Think about it for a second: How do you think you would react?

Although there's no way of knowing all the sources of this manganese that may be attributed in each particular case, I do now regularly see and recognize the disastrous result of these excesses and associated sensitivities in both children and adults. Our research has revealed that beyond food sources, we can also be exposed to manganese through such means as our water and combustion emissions. However, I believe it likely that in most cases the storing of excess manganese can be more attributed to the lack of iron in a person's diet and/or the lack of the bioavailability and absorption of iron due to dietary factors and other gut-related problems, than specifically to the high consumption of or other exposures to manganese. This is why at our Center, in addition to the manganese issues, we prefer to simultaneously address any gut and mal-absorption issues. No food or supplement in the world will be effective if you are not absorbing the nutrients in the first place.

I have seen the suspected culprits in manganese excesses be anything from toxic exposure (in the case of a welder), to the use of many soy baby formulas, to a low-iron diet coupled with excessive vitamin consumption. Wherever the excess comes from, it's important that you get rid of it! The best thing you can do for the issue for yourself and/or as a parent is to become a diligent food and product label reader. You will need published reference materials or at least our lists to identify generic food items that are relatively-high in manganese, however we have seen amazingly-high levels of manganese listed right on the labels of anything from baby foods and formulas, to popular breakfast cereals and many other processed foods, so pay strict attention! Our recommendation is that if the content for manganese is not shown on a label, then play it safe and either research it, or avoid it.

Since I practice as a Traditional Naturopath, a named "diagnosis" doesn't mean much to me. I have more of a tendency to look at symptoms and how and why they occur, than to have a need to give something a name or label. In my practice, I choose to use a form of evoked potential bio-feedback to try to detect bodily stress in response to an excess, and that's how I originally suspected the condition and syndrome. But quite frankly, no matter the result of any form of testing, if a person/child is exhibiting these recognizable symptoms, I'd go ahead and try the Protocol at any rate.

So instead of concentrating on any specific "diagnosis", just refer under our Frequently Asked Questions section to my list of some of the most common clinical symptoms of manganese overload and how they may relate to all kinds of diagnosis's and syndromes. There are sometimes more than these listed, but anyone presenting any or many of these in particular will put me on high alert.

The issue that is constantly raised and I believe obsessed over by many in the allopathic medical community and even in Autism groups, is how to precisely identify and quantify the presence of excess manganese in a manner acceptable to them using standard medical testing procedures. To this I respectfully respond, "Who cares?!" When the above-mentioned symptoms are present, why initially jump to expensive and invasive testing procedures and possibly to drugs? Why not just try the dietary Protocol for at least a short time and see what happens? Aside from the presence of any specific allergies, I am not aware of any possible side-effects from this type of dietary modification. Although I would highly suggest having the support of a health professional whenever possible, even parents at home can start this program independently and just see how it goes.

We have had both children and adult clients come to us who have elsewhere had metals testing done in the forms of blood work and/or hair analysis that do not seem to evidence any "excesses" of manganese. The problem with this limiting assumption is at least three-fold:

1. The problem we have theorized, which has been supported with plentiful historic third party research, is that the manganese sensitivity occurs most specifically within the brain chemistry, so neither blood nor hair testing alone will necessarily reveal and/or confirm this condition

2. We are talking here about individual sensitivity to manganese, and not a syndrome that can be applicable or susceptible to all children or adults. I often use the analogy of a person being allergic to a food such as peanuts: As one person could eat a pound of peanuts and have no ill effects and the next person may experience a violent allergic response to a minuscule exposure, it is obvious that the response produced by the peanuts is far more important in the equation than just the amount of peanuts that might be measured and quantified in one's body

3. There is much disagreement and conflicting information in nutritional and toxicological research fields as to what actual levels of ingestion and retention of manganese is even considered

safe above very trace amounts. We have found numerous studies internationally that have pointed to negative consequences suspected from manganese levels that are currently considered to be within acceptable standards. We certainly hope that our work will motivate more definitive research and reconsideration regarding this important matter

But as it turns out, there's more to it than just Manganese & Iron: "The Spinach Paradox"

Spinach happens to be one of the very first foods that demonstrated to us its ability to help trigger the stabilization of excess manganese and rapid reduction of unwanted symptoms in my child clients, however the wonder-leaf also became a point of temporary frustration for us due to a subsequent realization that at first seemed to be a potential contradiction in the logic of our already successful dietary Protocol. We have referred to this turning point in understanding as "The Spinach Paradox".

By the summer of 2008, we had a good deal of client cases under our belt and we were aggressively ramping up our efforts to get the word out to the medical and Autism research communities in order to attract help in dramatically advancing and expanding the work. One complaint that we were hearing over and over from parents was that we didn't have enough food items categorized on the diet to allow diverse enough meals for the whole family over extended periods of time.

It was true; at that time we had a fairly short listing of no more than a couple dozen foods on our two "eat" and "avoid" lists, and due to the fact that things seemed to be working so well despite our having so little available pertinent reference information, we had been extremely cautious about adding more process that didn't seem to be in any way broke? But still, we had to agree that we might have greater and more consistent compliance if we were able to add greater variety to the meal possibilities.

One day my brother Doug sat down at his computer to try to locate more foods that I might be able to recommend with confidence. Logical Internet searches involved lists of "foods that are highest in iron", and lists of "foods that are highest in manganese". He later described a particular day that resulted in so much confusion and frustration that he was literally afraid to bring the new data to my attention.

The concern arose when a particular search result located a list of foods that were considered to be "excellent sources of manganese", and he noticed that near the top of the list was one of our Protocol heroes – spinach. How was it possible that spinach, one of our first assumed trigger foods that put us on our path of discovery, was considered as good a source of dietary manganese, as it was of iron? I think he nearly had a heart attack. Was this revelation destined to throw our entire theory out the window? Were we now back to square one??

However, as our ongoing research has revealed to us, the answer as to why spinach "works" within the Protocol is more complicated than just its ability to simultaneously provide both minerals and then have the iron simply "win out" over the manganese. As we started researching the overall nutrient content of foods more completely, it became increasingly obvious that there are other factors that have influence on this important mineral balancing act such as certain vitamins and compounds present or absent in foods that tend to either enhance or inhibit iron absorption and utilization.

Our intent in this writing is not to over-complicate our food selection and rating process for you, so just know that the there are a number of underlying factors within the nutritional profiles of the foods taken into consideration, and therefore we suggest adhering to our food rating system in preference to any seeming contradictions that may result from simply searching, cross-referencing and contrasting lists of high-iron and high-manganese foods. Additional information will surely become available soon.

Spinach continues to have a net-positive effect in the whole process, however over time we have identified a number of foods that we feel are even superior for our purposes. But never the less, we will always be thankful to spinach in serving as one of the first heroes for the kids in our program. Popeye saves the day once again!

Potential Application and Effectiveness beyond ASD Cases

I, like many practitioners who work with ASD's, believe that less-severe symptoms associated with many diagnosis's of PDD-NOS, ADD, ADHD, Sensory Integration Disorder and others are all less pronounced expressions along the same Autism Spectrum, and therefore may share in this same dietary/nutritional imbalance that is producing various degrees of "brain fog" consequences.

As the majority of our clients seek our help for general wellness, and to a growing degree for help with ASD's, we have far less clinical experience with specific psychological issues. However, we have seen sufficient benefit from our Protocol with both children and adult clients to suggest that the same dietary links and imbalances that we have identified (the Menefe Syndrome) may be contributing factors in many other disorders that involve informational processing breakdowns in the brain.

So for physicians, other practitioners and therapists, this represents an additional consideration for trying this dietary modification therapy with patients who are dealing with such disorders as OCD, Tourette Syndrome, Chronic Depression, Generalized Anxiety Disorder, Bi-Polar/Schizophrenia and even Alzheimer's. Certainly no harm will be done, and if such cases are going to positively respond to these dietary changes, this "trigger" effect should result in some subjectively and objectively noticeable improvements in as little as 2-4 weeks of strict compliance, so this will not represent a very protracted or laborious experiment in exchange for the potential upside.

Now I know what many of you will be thinking when first reviewing the attached diet, because nearly all the parents say the same thing: You'll be wondering how you'll get your kids to eat these foods, right? I mean, "Don't all kids hate sweet potatoes and spinach"? The answer to this, as unbelievable as you may find it, is a big *NO*. The children (and the adults) almost to a person have all found themselves, once exposed to it, actually craving many of the iron-rich meats, veggies and fruits suggested on the diet. One 9-year-old I was discharging from regular monitoring after a few months was very concerned that since he was technically going off the program, whether he could still eat spinach because he "loved it so much". His Mom assured him that he could have it anytime he wanted it; something she never expected to say to her formerly vegetable-hating picky eater!

Trust me; most kids tend to adapt to the diet readily. And even if they don't at first – make them stay on it! You're the adult, and you get to make the choices. A few of the kids (like the one who only liked fast-food and cereals) threw some major tantrums and/or went a little hungry for a couple of days, but in the end they have virtually all come around to adapting to and enjoying the diet. Honestly, the biggest adaptation problem we have seen is with parents who are resistant at first to preparing breakfasts for the family that involve more than just pouring something out of a box, or lunches that aren't between two slices of bread. *We truly wish that we could make the diet even easier, but unless you are prepared and able to avoid the types of foods that have helped create the problem in the first place, you cannot have the expectation of achieving real and sustained improvements.*

Before putting people and especially children on lifelong courses of very serious and expensive drugs with very real potential for side-effects and/or into very expensive behavior modification programs, why not get the person on this high-iron/low-manganese Protocol and see if there is any positive result? The usual response time for the first significant changes to be noticed is quite rapid, and no one in this world is going to be damaged by a few weeks of this diet – in simple contrast to the prospect of starting on many prescription drugs where it often seems that potential side-effects can be as bad or worse than the targeted condition or disease itself.

One of the drawbacks to so many of the other dietary regimes I have reviewed that are designed to aid various conditions, is that they are quite difficult to maintain. They require a lot of portion control, specific shopping, very limited choice, and just forget about ever traveling or eating out! It usually also means making one meal for the affected child or adult and another meal for everyone else. The diet I am recommending will be wholesome, healthy, tasty, varied and satisfying for the whole family.

The "portion control" for this Protocol does not include anything measured in ounces except in the case of dairy and specific supplements that we might individually recommend. Neither do we include instructions on how many times a day to eat something in particular, or dictate any one food that you must eat. Truthfully I tried to do that at first because that type of strict regulation is far more readily accepted by the medical community at large, but it just didn't work as well, and I'm completely results oriented.

My standard instruction to parents is exactly this: ***"Every time your child wants something to eat, just make sure whenever possible that it's from one of our "Best Choices" columns"***. This includes breakfast, lunch, dinner AND snacks. If at first they only like a few things on the lists, then let them eat those foods – over and over. It always amuses me when I hear, "I love salmon" or "I love spinach" out of the mouth of a child (especially one who had little or no language skills before the dietary Protocol), but it just keeps happening.

So in summary, you'll find that the basics of the Protocol are just that – very basic. As I mentioned before, I honestly believe that one of the barriers to acceptance by most medical doctors (or even by the public in general) has been how simple and easy this actually is: Give the digestion system some support, increase bio-available iron consumption, enhance iron absorption and minimize manganese intake. Pretty simple isn't it? How can something as easy as balancing the iron and manganese levels in the body erase these horrible and debilitating symptoms? Answer again: *"I don't yet have every answer, but who cares as long as it works!"* This is a gift. Be grateful for it.

FREQUENTLY ASKED QUESTIONS

How do I know if my child is, or I am, a good candidate for this Protocol?

1. If any person is displaying associated symptoms and/or has been diagnosed anywhere along the Autistic Spectrum (PDD-NOS, ADD, ADHD, Sensory Integration Disorder, Asperger Syndrome, classic Autism, etc.) or has any other form of chronic psychological or behavioral issues, then it's worth a try. As this is just about "food", no one will be harmed in trying.

2. If the person in question in displaying any of these particular symptoms:

A. **Oversensitivity to sensory input:** This is first and foremost, and I have rarely seen anyone in our program who didn't display at least some of this. Sometimes it can be an overreaction to a single sensory source such as light, noise or certain sounds, but it's often from combinations of input. This can manifest in ways such as not wanting to be around other people (especially in a classroom, restaurant or shopping mall), flinching, squinting or watering eyes in bright light, intensely smelling everything from fabrics to foods (sometimes getting very offended by strong smells), to always complaining that they are "being yelled at". It can also induce claustrophobia and a tendency to physically strike out at anyone who gets too close. On the "touch" end, I've seen kids who refuse haircuts because they can't stand the way the little cut hairs "hurt" them, who can't stand wearing bedclothes, or who keep tearing off their clothes because of the little tags in the neck of a shirt. If your child is light or sound sensitive, hates going to the mall, doesn't like to go to the movies, constantly sniffs all his/her food or hates all the shirts with tags on them, you're probably looking at a case of sensory overload. Although it shows up in varying degrees, this is the most common of the issues and reflects the basis of the problem.

B. **"Extreme" Dreaming:** Frequent, horribly frightening and very realistic Technicolor nightmares that they have difficulty waking up from are quite common. Others might just dream very frequently and in extreme detail. Children often times don't voluntarily tell their parents about these dreams, but it will manifest in a kid who always wants to sleep with Mom and Dad, or at the very least can't sleep without a night light. Others tell long very-involved stories about the vivid dream they had the night before. At least 90% of the time these affected people tell me that the worst part of the dreams are that objects, people or quite commonly "demons" or other scary beasts, are "coming at them from everywhere", or that they are being "pounced on" or otherwise attacked. Another strange aspect of these dreams is that for some reason in many people, the syndrome seems to invoke some of the darker areas of the subconscious resulting in dreams that the person is actually ashamed of for even thinking.

C. **Impulsivity and/or "Blurting":** This can range from saying inappropriate things or acting out, all the way to violence – sometimes even extreme violence. A common statement to look for from older vocal children and adults is, "I know I shouldn't be doing that, but I just can't stop myself", which is often accompanied by tears of frustration or recriminations that they are "a bad person". It took me a long time to stop being shocked at some of the things children said to their parents or siblings, or sometimes even to me during office visits. These things range from the odd or inappropriate to incredibly sarcastic, cruel or lewd. I've had everything from kids who tell me how horrible their parents are, to those who started screaming and cursing at, or even hitting, their parent who was with them.

D. **"Scenario Building", or hearing voices in their head:** So common that it is nearly universal, is this "scenario building". It involves hearing your own voice (or sometimes someone else's) in your head making up wild stories and primarily-negative fantasies. In children (especially the younger ones) this manifests most often in fear and particularly in paranoia. They very often are afraid of other children, teachers, normally harmless animals, or of what they project someone may do to them – even their own parents. Some of the scenarios related to me by children have been absolutely chilling, and there have been some very shocked expressions on the faces of Moms who find out that their own beloved kids are afraid of them or their Fathers. It also shows up regularly as the "tall story teller" with a child who either wildly exaggerates or just commonly lies altogether. The thing to remember is that because of the high sensory input, this "tall tale" stuff is quite often not an exaggeration in their mind, but rather exactly as they remember it happening.

E. **Related Physical Symptoms and Especially Digestive Complaints:** Not always, but with enough regularity to definitely mention, I see that kids who fall into this category also have chronic stomach pains, diarrhea or constipation, rashes, eczema, allergies or asthma. Presenting with these symptoms alone I would not necessarily first consider our syndrome, but these often accompany the other more-recognizable ones.

Is this program expensive to take on?

In a word...no. Even with those clients who are able to travel to see us, we usually only recommend limited supplements, and the necessary food items can all be easily included on your family's usual shopping list. If you're not accustomed to eating anything beyond fast-food, then this will probably be somewhat more expensive for you. If you usually eat quality foods, then you probably won't notice a significant difference in your budget as the diet is mostly based on avoidance and substitution.

How difficult is this diet to follow? Can we still eat in restaurants?

The diet is actually relatively simple. No measuring or worrying about specific portions or searching for foods and ingredients you've never heard of, and the best part is that the diet will be healthy, nutritious and delicious for the whole family. There's no justification for having to make more than one meal for the whole gang – a real plus for busy parents. Although eating out can present a real wildcard, an occasional restaurant that offers decent quality food should not present much risk.

Do I have to eat the same foods as my child?

The best results we're witnessing here in Durango and hearing back from many of our home-based programs are consistently from the families that have *all family members eating by the SBP Diet guidelines.* **We can't stress the importance of this enough!** Trying to make different meals for various kids and adults in the same household is not only time consuming and overly complicated, but produces feelings of exclusion for those who are made to feel that they're being singled out for special treatment. If a child is to properly appreciate that this represents "healthier" eating choices for them, then how are they able to accept that their foods are somehow not good enough for the rest of the family? And also, if you keep junk food in your house, whether it's under your bed or on top of the fridge, your child will find it. Set a good and healthy example and eat by this diet as a family. Your positive attitude that the changes are "no big deal" will go a long way with your kids, and trust us here; Dad, Mom and everyone else will see that they feel better on the SBP Diet as well!

How do I get my picky-eater kid to eat healthier foods and go without a few favorite items?

Actually, it's probably much easier than you might think. Unlike adults who are set in their ways, once you show kids a better way to go, they generally grab onto the changed lifestyle with gusto. I have seen two-year-olds (and older) who walk around with open bags of raw spinach eating from it like another kid might with a bag of potato chips. Besides, it's not essential that you serve a large variety of foods in order for this process to start working. If the child initially only seems to like a limited number of food items on the diet, then let them eat just those for a little while. Many of the most beneficial foods can also be blended into "smoothies" that most kids don't have much problem with. Purees that mix meat and vegetables, or fruit and vegetables (not fruit with meat), can be very effective. I know some of this may sound a little far-fetched at first, but trust me - the kids usually do just fine. It's generally harder to change the habits of the parents than of the kids!

We are practicing vegetarians. Do have suggestions for us regarding this diet?

We continue to attempt to apologize in advance to our many adult friends out there who have adopted a vegetarian or vegan lifestyle not only for themselves, but attempt to likewise raise their children with such choices - many times from infancy. We surely can appreciate that choice, but best success with the SBP Diet is proving to be much slower if not nearly impossible in such cases due primarily to the challenges of getting enough protein and iron from the plant-source foods that we don't otherwise restrict in Phase 1 of the diet. As we try to remind people, we neither have the agenda nor desire to challenge or debate the validity of dietary choices in a family based on philosophical, cultural, religious, environmental or any other priorities. Ours is simply a mission of sharing information and education that people are willing to freely use or reject at their discretion. As they say, don't shoot the messenger! For example; the reality that our bodies are able to utilize a nutrient such as dietary iron obtained from animal foods much more efficiently than the iron contained in vegetables does not represent "our opinion", but a simple fact of biochemistry. The prospect for the anti-nutrient action of phytic acid/ phytate producing mineral depletion and resulting imbalances in our bodies is not our "opinion", but is instead a fact of nutritional science that has been well researched, studied and documented, but not adequately valued, reported or properly applied to human nutrition over many decades. Just do a little research on these important topics for yourself.

Some of these recommendations go against what I've been told or have come to believe. Is it really healthy for me or my family to eat this way?

Regardless of your prior education, assumptions, beliefs and resulting choices for your personal diet, we only ask for you to continue to look beyond a number of the food choices that have been marketed and pushed upon consumers over the last several decades, and to possibly reconsider the growing evidence, such as that being continually confirmed by the positive results from the SBP Diet, that maybe less than ideal nutritional needs of developing infants and young children (or even adults) can be and are being met with just *any* profile of desired foods. And please never feel that you have to just take our word for it: Just a little research and investigation on your part will reveal plentiful and mounting evidence that there are far more potential consequences for the function and wellness of the bodies of ourselves and our children than we've been led to believe for a long time now. Many researchers and the nutritionally educated are starting to get it, and there's a multitude of books, online writings and other resources that will supply you with added confirmation that people need to reeducate themselves about the dramatic benefits and consequences of their food choices.

How long should this take to see any results?

That's difficult to predict with any consistency as every case is certainly different, although we need to reinforce that the people who adhere most strictly to this Protocol will always see the fastest results. As a general rule, the younger (and smaller) the child, the quicker the parents usually see some results. In general – let us stress that – IN GENERAL, we are commonly seeing the first significant changes beginning somewhere within the first 15–30 days of strict and proper compliance.

Is it normal to experience ups & downs, good & bad days and other inconsistencies while on this diet?

Absolutely. As much as we would like to say that everyone sees progress in some uniform, cumulative and predictable manner, the majority of people see ups and downs that if not anticipated, may seem like setbacks or regression. The process can be very different for many due to individual sensitivities to the Menefe Syndrome and the particular severity and duration of the condition and unwanted symptoms. Setbacks almost always settle down within a couple of days, so stay with it!

Is it normal in the beginning that my child seems to still feel hungry after meals?

Many people quickly recognize that the SBP Diet reduces many of the carbohydrate foods that have commonly become large parts of the modern diet of many. The abrupt reduction of these foods is often associated with cravings and feelings of less fullness until your body efficiently adjusts to using higher percentages of protein and healthy fats as fuel and to alternate sources of fiber, in preference to all the breads, cereals and other low-value carbs that provide those accustomed feelings of "fullness", but may also promote weight issues, blood sugar irregularities and in the case of some foods, the specific nutritional imbalance that we have identified. Do quick calorie counts of a few meals and you'll be reassured that you're not starving anyone. Just do your best to be a little patient initially.

If my child's (or my) behavior or symptoms actually seem to get "worse", either immediately after starting the diet or several weeks into the diet, does that mean that the process is not working correctly?

We like to say that *any* resulting changes in symptoms and behavior are indications that you're making positive progress. It is important to understand that all we're doing here is substituting some foods for other foods, so here's our logic regarding the process that I think will make sense to you:

• Obviously the best and most desirable reaction and outcome will be rapid, progressive and cumulative improvements

• But another positive indicator and reaction may actually be a temporary worsening of some symptoms. If the Menefe Syndrome were not indeed present, then it would be more likely to notice absolutely nothing from the dietary changes

• Therefore, the WORST outcome we could expect would be to notice absolutely no changes, good or bad, over the entire process

What do I do regarding missing foods items that you don't have anywhere listed?

If a particular food item isn't listed and categorized, just don't eat it! Usually missing whole food items simply means that we have not yet been able to locate the nutritional information we need to properly rank them to our satisfaction. We ask people to appreciate that beyond the U.S., we have practitioners and families all around the world considering if this diet makes reasonable sense, and we therefore try our best to only refer to generic whole foods that much of the world will also have access and availability to. Packaged and otherwise processed foods will always represent unknown variables in the ways that they may influence your program dependent on such factors as the sources, ingredient quality and content, chemical content, GMO food content (a steadily increasing concern) and other and potentially undisclosed and unknown factors. Your best control is always to prepare meals with whole and organic foods whenever and wherever possible. When you can't always locate organic, then just do your best to buy from trusted sources. There are TONS of whole food items in the diet now, so please just do your best with these for the time being.

Isn't there some way to just make this diet "easier"?

We hear and acknowledge frustration from many that the SBP dietary suggestions seem for various reasons to be difficult to adopt, and we can understand their hopes that the process can somehow be made simpler. One of the initial observations and comments that we commonly hear is that "There's no way that my child will be able to eat this way because all his/her favorite foods are on your Don't Eat at All for Now lists." It's very important for those who feel that way to pause and try to recognize that there's an extremely good and self-evident reason for that predicament. It's not like we or others set out to see just how many of the favorite foods of children or adults we can deprive them of. There are powerful chemical reasons that many people feel quite literally "addicted" to certain foods, and just because someone craves a particular food is not sufficient validation of its nutritional value or necessity in their diet. Over the last several decades our poor eating habits and high consumption of processed foods has really taken us off a cliff, and we must now rebuild our knowledge and re-prioritize the importance of proper nutritional choices – especially for those very early in their lives. Remember that the SBP dietary recommendations are simply offered for you to try, or not try, along with our sincere hope that if you do elect to give it a solid effort, you will rapidly start seeing some confirmation that the process is benefiting the wellness of you, your child and the entire family, and that this will give you confidence that these lifestyle changes are well worth it in many ways.

How do we know when we should transition between the three "Phases" of the program?

Transitions from using only the Best Choices list foods to more on the Moderation lists should ALWAYS be done based on behavior and NEVER simply on the length of time on the Protocol. You cannot just say, "I've been on Phase 1 for 'X' number of weeks, so it's time to move to Phase 2". When your child is behaving and learning the way you would like them to, then and only then is the time to move on to the next Phase. As everyone is different, it's going to be up to you, your medical practitioners and therapists to judge the level of results and best transitions. Once you have moved on to Phase 3 we strongly believe that you'll appreciate that this represents an excellent dietary lifestyle to stay on indefinitely, but remember that if you see any signs of regression, you can always temporarily return to the more strict requirements of Phase 1 anytime you wish.

What about the use of medications & supplements along with this diet?

We at No Harm Foundation, and especially Dr. Shauna, are often asked about medications and nutritional supplements that we recommend or do not recommend. First and foremost, our goal is always to have the dietary changes do most of the work whenever possible, however we know that often there are other issues that children and adults are experiencing that the diet alone can not be expected to completely address. Please understand that as we are not medical doctors, we can in no way legally or even ethically advise you about the use or dosage of any prescription drugs. You will need to consult with your prescribing physicians for all such guidance. There are so many nutritional supplements available out there, yet with unpredictable availability (especially with international considerations), so it's rarely practical or even responsible for us to try to recommend generic supplementation for people to try to locate in their markets or even health food stores. There are superior and inferior brands and many other variables in your choices out there, and Shauna always prefers to keep supplements minimized and fairly customized to the individual case at any rate.

THE SPECTRUM BALANCE® PROTOCOL DIET
Revision: 141202

This is intended to replace all prior versions

Since foods form the cornerstone and most vital parts of this Protocol, pay particular attention to our relative rankings of the many food items that follow. Due to still expanding research, this is a growing yet incomplete list considering all the food choices out there, but this guide should easily give you enough options to create a variety of complete meals and snacks, and ones that the whole family will enjoy and benefit from nutritionally. If you are not prepared and ready to strictly follow these recommendations, then just wait until you are. *It is imperative to understand that an inadequate 50% compliance will in no way produce a 50% or more positive result, so treat this program very seriously if you wish to achieve any significant success.*

Now, please trust that we know what many of you will be thinking when first reviewing these lists…"What do you mean to not eat (…whatever). I've heard that it's very good for you!" Understand that the key here is that we are suggesting that you concentrate on eating certain foods and avoiding certain other foods because of their overall nutritional profiles and the ways that they might ease, perpetuate or aggravate the symptoms present. Therefore we suggest adhering to our food rating system regardless of any seeming contradictions with more "conventional" thought out there. Once balance is restored in the body and ongoing dietary responsibility is practiced in the future, many foods that may be your favorites will return to being fine to consume, at least in moderation. If you don't see a particular food item in any of our categories, it's because we haven't yet been able to locate sufficient information to classify it with any confidence. The lists will expand as further research is completed, so the Golden Rule for now is…*If you don't see a food listed, then please just avoid it!*

Our intent with this simple guide is to not over-complicate the food selection and rating process, so just know that there are a good number of underlying factors taken into consideration when ranking these foods with specific regard to their influence on an all-important nutrient balancing act, such as certain vitamins and compounds being present or absent that tend to either enhance or inhibit nutrient absorption and utilization. We have taken into account both nutrient as well as "anti-nutrient" properties of foods in creating this unique reference.

The processing and packaging of foods always has negative impact on their nutritional content, so whole foods and *fresh* juicing are always preferred. Whenever possible, try to only steam your cooked vegetables and avoid microwaving. Only *un-sulfured* dried fruits should be used where indicated. Also remember that we are rating foods with the assumption that you're preparing most meals from home. Be aware that restaurant and fast-foods will be of unknown and varying nutritional quality and therefore may produce suboptimal results for you.

We're making absolutely no philosophical, cultural, religious, environmental or other judgments about these foods, and you'll certainly need to take into planning any foods that you or your children have known allergies or other sensitivities to. Just do your best to use this ranking system to plan meals using those food items that you can locate and are agreeable with. With a little creativity and practice, we're sure you'll find plenty on these lists that your child and the rest of the family will be happy to eat – ***and most important, it will all be worth it!***

Most Important Factors:

You will find that the foods groups that follow are divided into three very important categories:

"Best Choices" – These are the foods that you will want to utilize in planning your meals whenever and wherever possible. Any positive results that you will achieve from these dietary changes will be in direct proportion to how well you comply with these recommendations. The food items in this category reflect our best suggestions that will allow you to hopefully notice initial results within the shortest time-frame.

"Eat Only in Moderation" – The primary purpose of this second column is to offer you a greater assortment of foods for your meal planning, but their value in the dietary therapy is considered to be mostly "neutral", in that our expectation is not that they will be especially beneficial in your overall program, but more that they will not be detrimental in your program. A good rule of thumb: Try to eat a mix of at least 2-3 portions (by volume) of Best Choices items to every 1 portion (by volume) of Eat Only in Moderation items.

"Don't Eat at All for Now!" – Just what it says, and this is by far the most important classification of our food instructions to strictly comply with. ***If you do not avoid the foods in this column virtually completely during at least the first Phase of this dietary program, then you run the risk of negating much of the progress being achieved.*** Taking one step forward only to take one step backward will help no one and will drastically reduce your patience and potential with this Protocol.

It is important to realize and appreciate that unlike many highly-specific and potentially-lifetime dietary protocols that are recommended in support of many Spectrum Disorders, our Spectrum

Balance® Protocol is designed to produce certain primary changes and bring greater equilibrium in the body, and once positive response is experienced the diet will transition to being less stringent. As reinforced above, it is of the utmost importance that you maintain strict compliance in the beginning, however we generally see your initial and long term maintenance plan being broken into three "Phases" that will progress according to your own body's response and rate of improvement. ***Don't be frustrated by any temporary ups and downs in your progress!!***

Phase 1: Typically the first 4-6 weeks on the program are the most important to the pace of your progress, and during this time we ask that you eat foods predominately from the "Best" columns with all others from the "Moderation" columns. If you do not have a healthcare practitioner helping you monitor your program, then you will want to strictly stay in Phase 1 as long as you are seeing building progress.

Phase 2: Typically the remainder of at least your first 3 months on the program. Although we ask that you always consider the Best Choices that we recommend for the vast majority of your dietary needs, it will become less imperative that you completely avoid all foods in our "Don't Eat" category. Again, you alone set and control the pace of your progress, but a little "cheating" here and there in Phase 2 should not be of any major consequence. ***Always base these transitions on changes in behavior.***

Phase 3: Once you have been able to see how your body is reacting to the dietary changes over the first 3 months, most people are able to start eating with more balance within all three categories, but you should always remember what your body has told you about what's best for you and continue to eat in a more healthy pattern in order to preserve your highest level of wellness. Continue to avoid grains and legumes and minimize consumption of dairy on an ongoing basis (see Phase 3 Diet attached).

So please do your best to be patient and compliant with the process and know that if a "favorite food" just happens to appear in our "Don't Eat at All for Now" category, you may only be asked to live without it temporarily with the exception of a few types of foods that just might never work positively with your body no matter how much you may like their tastes. There are plenty of great foods available out there so try your best not to focus on the minority you should avoid in order to stay healthier! Always be mindful of the date at the top of this document due to the fact that we make changes and updates as often as practical. Our clients are always welcome to check back with us and we'll be happy to furnish anyone with an updated version if available.

Note to our vegetarian friends: Please be aware that those who have chosen a vegetarian or vegan lifestyle for yourselves and/or your children will have a special challenge with this program as you review our restrictions on most of the grains, soy & legumes and nuts that serve as staples for most non-meat and non-dairy eaters. Because the absorption of meat-source iron (heme iron) tends to accelerate progress with this Protocol to a far greater degree than plant-based iron (non-heme iron), vegetarians will be at a disadvantage. Just a fact.

FIRST: YOUR "COMPLETELY AVOID" LIST

Processed Foods – Eat whole foods whenever possible and avoid or at very least minimize eating processed and pre-packaged foods. If all you have to do is pour it out of a bag or box, add liquid and stir, you can be pretty sure it's full of chemicals. This is not just a SBP Diet rule, but a general rule of thumb for good health.

Artificial Sweeteners – Completely avoid ALL of them. The pink, the blue, the yellow, and become an effective food label reader to keep you and your kids from ingesting these substances in processed foods. Be aware that many times there are also artificial sweeteners hiding in chewing gums, toothpastes, drink mixes, etc.

Processed Sugars – Avoid all processed sweeteners and especially **high-fructose corn syrup** (HFCS), which is commonly found in processed foods. Stay with sparing use of natural sweeteners and herbals such as Stevia.

Grains & Legumes – Do your best to avoid all possible. Watch your processed food labels closely because wheat and soy ingredients are hiding everywhere. **No soy milks for anyone and no soy formulas for infants.**

Cow's Milk – We make cautionary allowances for limited use of some dairy foods unless you have known contraindicating issues. Yes, unprocessed dairy can be superior to processed, but please avoid drinking all milks for the time being and see how the changes benefit your health and the way that you feel.

Multi-vitamin Supplements – It's best to avoid all of them for now. Many of these contain vitamins and minerals that may be able to build up in cumulative concentrations within the body that may actually contribute to the problems. Often when people start adding up the numbers, they find that they're actually consuming nutrients at hundreds of percent of requirements and recommended intakes. Place higher reliance on getting more of your nutritional needs from your foods as compared to supplements. Saves money too!

GMOs (Genetically Modified Foods) - *Do everything you can to avoid GMO (genetically modified) foods!* In simplest terms, a GMO is a crop that has been genetically modified to produce a desired trait it currently doesn't have, such as being insect resistant. Although foods like soy and corn are disallowed on the Protocol anyway, there is more and more use of GMOs in tomatoes, papaya, and squash which are allowed. Do your best to buy organic for those products!

SPECTRUM BALANCE® PROTOCOL DIET
Revision: 141202

Food Categories & Relative Ratings
Food Items are Listed Alphabetically within their Categories

FRUITS – Be reasonable about servings of fruits due to sugar considerations

Best Choices	Eat Only in Moderation	Don't Eat at All for Now!
Acerola	Apples & Applesauce	Bananas
Apricots	Avocado	Blackberries
Cantaloupe Melon	Casaba Melon	Blueberries
Cherries – Black	Cherries – Red & white	Boysenberries
Clementines, Cuties	Cranberries – Raw, dried,	Coconut - Raw or dried
Currants – Black	sauce	Elderberries
Gooseberries	Currants - Zante	Grapes
Grapefruit – Pink, red,	Dates	Pineapple
white	Figs	Raisins
Guava	Nectarines	Raspberries
Honeydew Melon	Oranges	Strawberries
Kiwi	Peaches	
Lemons	Pears	
Limes	Pomegranate	
Mango	Prunes	
Papaya (non-GMO)		
Passion Fruit		
Plums		
Tangerines		
Watermelon		

JUICES & OTHER DRINKS - Be mindful of the sugar content of fruit juices!

Best Choices	Eat Only in Moderation	Don't Eat at All for Now!
Pure water – Maintain hydration with adequate water intake! Apricot Black Cherry Carrot Cranberry Grapefruit Guava Mango Papaya (non-GMO) Tangerine	Almond Milks - Original, vanilla or chocolate Orange Pear Sparkling water – Can be flavored with Stevia Tomato (non-GMO) Vegetable Juice	Apple Coconut Milk and Coconut Water Coffee Grape Pineapple Pomegranate Prune Rice Milk Soft Drinks – Regular or diet Soy Milk Teas – None for now

GREENS

Best Choices	Eat Only in Moderation	Don't Eat at All for Now!
Chinese Cabbage (Bok Choy) Collard Greens Dandelion Kale Lettuce – Butter, Red, Romaine Mustard Greens Swiss Chard Turnip Greens Watercress	Arugula Beet Greens Cabbage – All common types Fennel - Bulb, greens Onions/Scallions Radicchio Sauerkraut Spinach	Chrysanthemum Greens Endive Lettuce - Iceberg

VEGETABLES

Best Choices	Eat Only in Moderation	Don't Eat at All for Now!
Asparagus Broccoli Brussels Sprouts Carrots Cauliflower Celery Jerusalem Artichoke Peppers – Banana Peppers – Bell (red, orange, yellow) Peppers – Hot Chili Peppers – Pasilla Pumpkin Squash – Butternut Squash – Zucchini Sweet Potatoes (not the same as True "Yams")	Artichokes Cabbage – All common types Cucumbers Eggplant Jicama Leeks Olives Onions/Scallions Parsnips Pickles Peppers – Ancho Peppers – Bell (green) Peppers – Green Chili (canned) Peppers – Jalapeno Peppers – Serrano Radish Rhubarb Spinach Squash – Acorn Squash – Crookneck Squash – Spaghetti Squash – Summer varieties Tomatillos Tomatoes - All (non-GM) Tomato Sauce & Paste Turnips Water Chestnuts	Beets Cassava Corn – White & yellow Green Beans Mushrooms Okra Peas - Green Potatoes – All (white, gold, French fried, hashed, etc.) Rutabagas Seaweed Yams (True "Yams" are not the same as Sweet Potatoes, but are not common in the U.S.)

BEANS/ LEGUMES - Avoid all you can right now for best progress

Best Choices	Eat Only in Moderation	Don't Eat at All for Now!
None are Best Choices for now!	None are Best Choices for now!	Adzuki Black Beans Fava Beans (Broadbeans) Garbanzo Beans (Chickpeas) Green Beans Kidney Beans Lentils Lima Beans Miso Mung Beans Navy Beans Peanuts (yes,"legumes" not nuts) Peas – Green Pinto Beans Refried Beans Soy Beans & Soy Products Tofu White Beans

*Note regarding the Herbs & Spices below: We have simplified the following section by only separating herbs and spices into "Allowed" and "Don't Eat at All for Now" classifications. The Allowed choices can all be regularly used as long as an item does not constitute a main part of a meal, and all others should be avoided completely at least until Phase 3. Organic, garden grown, freeze dried and minimally processed versions of herb and spices are always preferred. **As always, if you do not see a particular food item listed, then assume that we have not yet found sufficient information to rank it with confidence and please just avoid it for now!**

HERBS & SPICES - Fresh or freeze-dried are superior to powered or with added salt

Best Choices	Eat Only in Moderation	Don't Eat at All for Now!
Basil	Salt – Celtic, Sea Salts,	Allspice
Bay Leaf	other natural forms only	Cardamom
Capers	Tarragon	Celery Seed
Chili Powder	Thyme	Cinnamon
Chives		Cloves
Coriander (Cilantro)		Cumin
Dill Weed		Curry Powder
Garlic – Fresh, freeze dried		Fennel Seed
		Garlic – Powered or salted
Ginger – Fresh, freeze dried		Ginger – Powdered
		Lemon Grass
Marjoram		Mustard Seed
Mint - Spearmint, Peppermint		Nutmeg
		Pepper – Black or white
Oregano		Poppy Seed
Paprika		Saffron
Parsley		Salt – All processed "table" versions
Pepper – Red or Cayenne		Savory
Rosemary		Turmeric
Sage		

MEATS & POULTRY – Locate nitrate-free processed meats such as sausages

Best Choices	More Best Choices	Don't Eat at All for Now!
Bacon (Pig-non nitrate) Beef – Grass Feed organic preferred Beef Liver Bison - Grass Feed organic preferred Chicken - Meat with skin is best Chicken Liver Cornish Game Hen Deer Duck Ham (non nitrate)	Elk Goat Lamb Pheasant Pork (pasture raised) Quail Rabbit Turkey – Meat, ground, turkey sausage, turkey bacon	Hot Dogs/ Franks – Beef & pork

FISH & SHELLFISH - Wild caught is always preferred over farm raised

Best Choices	Eat Only in Moderation	Don't Eat at All for Now!
Catfish Eel Halibut Lobster Mackerel Mahi Mahi Octopus Salmon – Atlantic, Chinook, Coho, Sockeye Sardines Squid Shrimp Tuna – Fresh preferred over canned (avoid soy broth) Whitefish	Anchovy Cod – Atlantic or Pacific Crab – Mixed species Grouper Monkfish Orange Roughy Oysters Pollock Scallops Sea Bass Snapper Tilapia Trout Yellow Tail	Clams Shark Swordfish

NUTS & SEEDS - Avoid all for the time being for best progress

Best Choices	Eat Only in Moderation	Don't Eat at All for Now!
None are Best Choices for now!	None are Best Choices for now!	Almonds Almond Butter Black Walnuts Cashews Cashew Butter Chestnuts Chia Flaxseed Hazelnuts Macadamia Peanuts Peanut Butter Pecans Pine Nuts (Pinion) Pumpkin Seeds (kernels or whole) Sesame Kernels (dried) Sesame Seeds Soybeans (roasted or other) Sunflower Seeds (kernels or whole) Walnuts

*Regarding use of the Dairy items below: Because of general health considerations more than because of Spectrum Balance® considerations, we caution against making dairy foods a significant portion of **anyone's** diet. However we are not of the belief that small inclusions of dairy in the diet of lactose tolerant individuals will result in the negative impact that we see from the consumption of larger quantities. All dairy items should only be eaten in moderation using the following simple guideline: **Eat no more than 1 oz. in total dairy over an entire day, and ideally not every day.** The reason that more cheeses are allowed where milks are not, is that it is far easier and realistic to measure and eat a single ounce of cheese in a meal than it is to drink only an ounce or so of milk.

DAIRY & EGGS

Best Choices	Eat Only in Moderation*	Don't Eat at All for Now!
Butter – Grass fed (organic) is preferred Eggs (free range preferred)	Cheese – American Cheese – Blue Cheese – Cheddar Cheese – Cottage Cheese – Feta Cheese – Mozzarella Cheese – Mexican Anejo Cheese – Monterrey Cheese – Muenster Cheese – Provolone Cheese – Ricotta Cheese – Romano Cheese – Swiss Cream Cheese Goat Cheese Sour Cream Yogurt – Goat Milk	Cheese – Parmesan Cow Milk Cow Milk – Chocolate, flavored Egg Substitutes Goat Milk Yogurt – Cow Milk Yogurt – Coconut Milk Yogurt – Soy

GRAINS, FLOURS & NOODLES - Avoid all you can right now for best progress

Best Choices	Eat Only in Moderation *	Don't Eat at All for Now!
None are Best Choices for now!	*** Although these choices are preferred to other options, we strongly suggest that you concentrate on recipes that transition your tastes and lifestyle away from reliance on baked goods and grain foods.** Arrowroot Carob Flour Sweet Potato Flour Tapioca – Pearled & Flour	Almond Flour Amaranth Barley Buckwheat Bulgur Coconut Flour Corn Flour – White & Yellow Corn Meal – White & Yellow Couscous Kamut Macaroni Millet Noodles – Egg & Spinach Noodles – Rice, Soba, Somen Oats, Oat Flour & Oat Bran Polenta Quinoa Rice – Brown, White Rice Flour & Bran – Brown Rice Flour & Bran – White Rye Flour Soy Flour Spaghetti Spelt Wheat Flour & Bran – All Wild Rice

BREADS - Avoid all you can right now for best progress

Best Choices	Eat Only in Moderation	Don't Eat at All for Now!
None are Best Choices!	None are good choices!	Bagels Biscuits Cornbread English Muffin – White & wheat French Bread Oat/Oat Bran Bread Pita – White & wheat Pumpernickel Rice Bran Rye Bread Spelt Bread Tortillas – Corn & flour Wheat Bread – Whole, bran, germ

BREAKFAST CEREALS - Applies to both generic & brand name products

Best Choices	Eat Only in Moderation	Don't Eat at All for Now!
None are Best Choices!	None are good choices! Avoid all cereals for best results	All processed & sugared cereals Corn flakes - Unsweetened Corn grits – White or Yellow Cream of rice Cream of wheat Millet – Puffed, cooked Oatmeal or oat bran cereals Rice – Puffed, unsweetened Wheat cereals - All

OILS, CONDIMENTS & COOKING

Due to the fact that we suggest heavily restricting the use of grains and flours, "baked goods" won't be a significant part of your diet. If you're baking with only the limited approved food items, baker's yeast can be used in very small amounts as long as you're not currently dealing with Candida or other yeast excess health issues.

Best Choices/ Allowed	Use Only in Moderation	Don't Eat at All for Now!
Butter	Almond Oil	Bacon Grease
Coconut Oil	Avocado Oil	Butter Substitutes
Cod Liver Oil	Baker's Yeast	Canola Oil
Flaxseed Oil (but do	Baking Powder	Lard
not use for cooking)	Baking Soda	Margarine – Regular
Olive Oil	Cream of Tartar	Margarine – Soy
Pepper – Red or Cay-	Horseradish	Palm Oil
enne	Ketchup – Low sugar	Peanut Oil
Salt – Celtic , Sea Salts	Mayonnaise – Natural	Pepper – Black or White
Vinegar – Balsamic is	Mustard	Rice Bran Oil
best	Pickle Relish	Safflower Oil
	Sesame Oil	Salt – Table
	Vinegar – Cider or Red	Shortening – Lard or
	Wine	Vegetable
	Worcestershire Sauce	Soy Sauce – All (Tamari)
		Soybean Oils
		Sunflower Oil
		Vegetable Oil – Canola or
		Corn

SWEETENERS & FLAVORING – Decrease your reliance on all sweeteners!

Best Choices	Use Only in Moderation	Don't Eat at All for Now!
Stevia - Herbal sweetener, also available in many flavors	Brown Sugar Carob – Unsweetened Honey Vanilla Extract	Agave (use Honey instead) Any and all artificial sweeteners Maple syrup Molasses White processed sugar - All forms

SNACKS & TREATS

Best Choices	Eat Only in Moderation	Don't Eat at All for Now!
Celery or carrot sticks Fresh fruit or veggie chunks from Best Choices list Freeze-dried or dehydrated fruits from Best Choices list Jerky, Pemmican (nitrate-free) Sweet Potato Chips - Natural	Fresh fruit or veggie chunks from Moderation list Freeze-dried or dehydrated fruits from Moderation list Mozzarella cheese sticks Tapioca pudding (no artificial sweeteners)	Cookies Corn Chips Crackers – Too many types to categorize accurately Graham Crackers Nuts Popcorn Pork Rinds Potato Chips Pretzels Raisins Rice Cakes Sugar Candies Tortilla Chips

THE SPECTRUM BALANCE® PROTOCOL
PHASE 3: Lifestyle Dietary Recommendations
Revision: 141202

Once you or your medical/therapy support personnel believe that you have attained and stabilized your goals using the primary Spectrum Balance® dietary modifications, we now want to give you our best recommendations for maintaining and building upon your achievements. Congratulations on teaching yourself valuable lessons that you'll be able to use to help keep you and your family feeling their best over a lifetime. Proper nutrition is the foundation of sustained health and wellness, so please don't fall back into the poor eating patterns that rob your body and brain of their unlimited potential. *Phase 3 represents a "lifestyle" eating and nutritional pattern; not a temporary "diet"!*

We'd really love to be able to tell you that you can now just go back to eating the same as you did previously, but over time we're seeing so much better prolonged and sustained success and general wellness with the ongoing practice of continuing to minimize or even avoid altogether just a minority of the multitude of food choices available to us. As everyone has different levels of sensitivity to the anti-nutrients and mineral imbalances that we address with the SBP Diet, pay special attention to how you feel as you begin making any changes in your program and watch closely for what your body tells you about any foods you resume eating that start negatively affecting the way you feel.

The good news is that you now have the knowledge to recognize problems early on and to use the foods you're eating to keep control over them. *Remember that you can always temporarily return to the more strict requirements of the SBP Phase 1 Diet anytime that you wish.*

So here are some guidelines to help keep you on track toward feeling better and better.

The Most Important Factors:

Remember that because processed and packaged foods will always be more likely to contain unwanted and even undisclosed ingredients we have concern for, we will still recommend that you continue to make whole foods and home prepared meals the greatest portion of your diet. Avoid overcooking and especially avoid microwaving your foods in order to preserve their best nutrient values. As always, you'll certainly need to take into account any foods that you or your children have known allergies or other sensitivities to when planning your meals using the following lists.

You will find that the large majority of our food choices for your Phase 3 plan are now divided into only two important categories:

"Best Choices" – These are the foods that you will want to utilize in planning your meals whenever and wherever possible. Any positive results that you have achieved and will continue to achieve from these dietary changes will be a direct function of how well you stay with these recommendations. You'll find now that fewer of your favorite foods will continue to be restricted.

"Continue to Minimize or Avoid" – We consider these to be the foods that promote the imbalances in your body that you've worked so hard to stabilize, so please continue to minimize or even avoid eating them altogether for best continued results. Where appropriate, we've made specific comments within the columns to warn you of the worst of the worst choices.

Reminder to our vegetarian friends: Please be aware that those of you who have chosen a vegetarian or vegan lifestyle for yourselves and/or your children are still advised to keep your consumption of legumes (especially soy), grains (especially wheat) and nuts as a much smaller portion of your total diet in comparison to your intake of fresh fruits and vegetables. Yes, the sprouting, fermenting and soaking of these seed-based foods will reduce some of the anti-nutrient content and their potential to promote mineral imbalances and deficiencies, but to unknown, unmeasurable and inconsistent degrees, so please take care.

THIS IS YOUR BASIC *"CONTINUE TO AVOID"* LIST

If we are able to impress upon you anything toward your journey to greater health from this point forward, it would be to continue to avoid all of the following. It's very common when people take a first look at our Spectrum Balance® Protocol Diet, that their first words are, "Oh no, many of my (or my child's) favorite foods are on your avoid lists!" Of course there's a very good reason for this. Our eating patterns that have been formed and driven by cravings produced by both natural and artificial chemical compounds present in many of our foods are greatly contributing to the weakening of our bodies and to the disruption of the wellness of society in general. So please continue to avoid…

Processed Foods – Continue to eat whole foods whenever possible and to minimize your consumption of processed and prepackaged foods. If all you have to do is pour it out of a bag or box, add water and stir, you can be pretty sure it's full of fillers and chemicals. Faster and cheaper – you bet, but poor choices for optimal wellness for sure. This is not just a "SBP rule", but a general rule of thumb for good health.

Artificial Sweeteners – Continue to avoid ALL of them - the pink, the blue, the yellow and continue being an effective food label reader in order to keep you and your children from ingesting these substances in processed foods and drinks. Also be aware that many times there are also artificial sweeteners hiding in chewing gums, toothpastes, drink mixes, etc.

Processed Sugars – Stay away from white table sugars, high-fructose corn syrup (HFCS) and as many other processed sweeteners as you are able. And again, a major point of control over this factor is to minimize your consumption of processed, packaged, ready-to-eat foods.

Soy & Other Legumes – Do your best to continue to avoid all legumes in your regular diet. Watch those processed food labels closely because soy ingredients are hiding everywhere and even show up in canned fish and other meats. Avoid soy milks for anyone and soy formulas for infants. Soy tends to be very high in both manganese and phytic acid content, and statistics show that in excess of 90% of the soy available in the U.S. results from genetically modified (GMO) crops, which just adds another reason to locate and rely on superior sources of protein and fiber.

Wheat & Other Grain Foods – The more we understand wheat and other grains through our own work and the work of others, the more our concerns build regarding the large amounts of phytochemicals and anti-nutrients we are regularly ingesting due to our strong addictions to these foods. Gluten-containing grains only represent one part of the complex problem. So very many people are reporting back to us that they just feel so much better when they continue to eliminate grains from their diets. Again… watch those packaged foods, because wheat ingredients are quite prevalent and you'll be amazed when you really start reading labels.

GMO & Modified Oil Products – Try to avoid all foods of known genetically modified origin and those that contain unnatural trans fats labeled as "shortening" and "hydrogenated", or "partially hydrogenated vegetable oil". Do your own research on these menaces to health.

Multi-vitamin Supplements – It's best to continue to avoid these unless you have received specific recommendations from someone trained in nutrition, and they will most likely also prefer that you supplement with specific and isolated nutrients at any rate. Many broad spectrum products contain a number of minerals and various other compounds that have the potential to build in cumulative concentrations within the body and can produce or contribute to the problem. Often when people put all their supplements together and start adding up the numbers, they find that they're actually consuming hundreds of percent of recommended daily values. Particularly avoid any supplements that include manganese. We get plenty of it from our fresh fruits and vegetables.

FRUITS – Be reasonable about servings of fruits due to sugar considerations

Best Choices	More Best Choices!	Continue to Minimize or Avoid
Acerola	Guava	Limit your consumption of:
Apricots	Honeydew Melon	
Apples & Applesauce	Kiwi	
Avocado	Lemons	Blueberries
Bananas	Limes	Pineapple
Blackberries	Mango	
Boysenberries	Nectarines	
Cantaloupe Melon	Oranges	
Casaba Melon	Papaya (non GMO)	
Cherries – Black, red & white	Passion Fruit	
Clementines, Cuties	Peaches	
Coconut	Pears	
Cranberries – Raw, dried, sauce	Plums	
Currants – Black, Zante	Pomegranate	
Dates	Prunes	
Elderberries	Raisins	
Figs	Raspberries	
Grapefruit – Pink, red & white	Strawberries	
Grapes	Tangerines	
	Watermelon	

JUICES & OTHER DRINKS – Be mindful of the sugar content of fruit juices!

Best Choices	More Best Choices!	Continue to Minimize or Avoid
Pure water – Maintain hydration with adequate water intake! Almond Milks - Original, vanilla or chocolate Apricot Black Cherry Carrot Coconut Water (not "Milk") Cranberry Grapefruit Guava Mango Orange	Papaya (non-GMO) Pear Pomegranate Prune Sparkling water flavored with plain or flavored Stevia Tangerine Teas – Herbals Tomato	Limit your consumption of: Apple Juice Coconut Milk Coffee Grape Pineapple Soft Drinks – Health store quality Teas – Black & Green Vegetable Juice Continue to avoid completely: Rice Milk Soft Drinks – Artificial sweeteners Soy Milk (*NONE!*)

GREENS

Best Choices	More Best Choices!	Continue to Minimize or Avoid
Arugula Beet Greens Cabbage – All common types Chinese Cabbage (Bok Choy) Collard Greens Dandelion Fennel (bulb, greens) Kale Lettuce – Butter, Red, Romaine	Mustard Greens Onions/Scallions Radicchio Sauerkraut Spinach Swiss Chard Turnip Greens Watercress	Chrysanthemum Greens Endive Lettuce - Iceberg

VEGETABLES

Best Choices	More Best Choices!	Continue to Minimize or Avoid
Artichokes	Peppers – Hot Chili	Cassava
Asparagus	Peppers – Jalapeno	Corn – White & yellow
Beets	Peppers – Pasilla	Peas – Green
Broccoli	Peppers – Serrano	Peppers – Bell (Green)
Brussels Sprouts	Pickles	Potatoes – All (white,
Cabbage – Common	Pumpkin	gold, French fried,
types	Radish	hashed, etc.)
Carrots	Rhubarb	Seaweed
Cauliflower	Rutabagas	Yams ("True Yams" are
Celery	Spinach	not the same as Sweet
Cucumbers	Squash – Acorn	Potatoes, but are not
Eggplant	Squash – Butternut	commonly found in the
Jerusalem Artichoke	Squash – Crookneck	U.S.)
Jicama	Squash – Spaghetti	
Leeks	Squash – Summer vari-	
Mushrooms	eties	
Okra	Squash – Zucchini	
Olives	Sweet Potatoes (not the	
Onions/Scallions	same as	
Parsnips	"True Yams")	
Peppers – Ancho	Tomatillos	
Peppers – Banana	Tomatoes - All (non-	
Peppers – Bell (Red,	GMO)	
orange, yellow)	Tomato Sauce / Paste	
Peppers – Green Chili	(organic, non -GMO)	
(canned)	Turnips	
	Water Chestnuts	

BEANS/ LEGUMES

Best Choices		Continue to Minimize or Avoid
None are best choices! Avoid all possible for your best long-term results		Black Beans Fava Beans (Broadbeans) Green Beans Kidney Beans Lentils Lima Beans Mung Beans Navy Beans Peanuts (yes, "legumes" not nuts) Peas – Green Pinto Beans Refried Beans White Beans **Continue to avoid completely:** Adzuki Beans Garbanzo Beans (Chickpeas) Miso Soy Beans & all Soy Products Tofu

HERBS & SPICES - Fresh or freeze-dried are superior to powered or with added salt

Best Choices	More Best Choices!	Continue to Minimize or Avoid
Allspice Basil Bay Leaf Capers Celery Seed Chili Powder Chives Coriander (Cilantro) Cumin Curry Powder Dill Weed Fennel Seed Garlic – Fresh, bulb Ginger – Fresh Lemon Grass Marjoram	Mint - Spearmint, Peppermint Mustard Seed Nutmeg Oregano Paprika Parsley Pepper – Black or white Pepper – Red or Cayenne Poppy Seed Rosemary Sage Salt – Celtic, Sea, natural forms Savory Tarragon Thyme	Limit your consumption of: Cardamom Cinnamon Cloves Garlic – Powdered or salted Ginger – Powdered Saffron Salt – Processed "table" versions Turmeric

MEATS & POULTRY - Locate nitrate-free processed meats, such as sausages

Best Choices	More Best Choices!	Continue to Minimize or Avoid
Bacon (Pasture raised, non-nitrite) Beef – Grass Feed organic preferred Beef Liver Bison - Grass Feed organic preferred Chicken - Meat with skin is best Chicken Liver Cornish Game Hen Deer	Duck Elk Goat Ham Lamb Pheasant Pork (Pasture raised) Quail Rabbit Turkey – Meat, sausage, bacon	Hot dogs - beef and pork

FISH & SHELLFISH – Wild caught is always preferred to farm raised

Best Choices	More Best Choices!	Continue to Minimize or Avoid
Anchovy Catfish Clams Cod – Atlantic or Pacific Crab – Mixed species Eel Grouper Halibut Lobster Mackerel Mahi Mahi Monkfish Octopus Orange Roughy Oysters Pollock	Salmon – Atlantic, Chinook, Coho Sockeye Sardines Scallops Sea Bass Shrimp Snapper Squid Tilapia Trout Tuna – Fresh preferred over canned (avoid soy broth) Yellow Tail Whitefish	Shark Swordfish

*Regarding use of Dairy items below: Because of general health considerations more than because of Spectrum Balance® considerations, we caution against making dairy foods a significant portion of **anyone's** diet. However we are not of the belief that small inclusions of dairy in the diet of lactose tolerant individuals will result in the negative impact that we see from the consumption of larger quantities. All dairy items should only be eaten in moderation using the following simple guideline: **Eat no more than 1 oz. in total dairy over an entire day, and ideally not every day.** The reason that more cheeses are allowed where milks are not, is that it is far easier and realistic to measure and eat a single ounce of cheese in a meal than it is to drink only an ounce or so of milk.

DAIRY & EGGS

Best Choices	Eat Only in Moderation	Continue to Minimize or Avoid
Butter – Grass fed (organic) is preferred Eggs – Free Range preferred	Cheese – American Cheese – Blue Cheese – Cheddar Cheese – Cottage Cheese – Feta Cheese – Mexican Anejo Cheese – Monterrey Cheese – Mozzarella Cheese – Muenster Cheese – Parmesan Cheese – Provolone Cheese – Ricotta Cheese – Romano Cheese – Swiss Cream Cheese Goat Milk & Cheese - Raw Sour Cream Yogurt – Cow Milk Yogurt – Goat Milk	Limit your consumption of: Cow Milk - Raw Continue to avoid completely: Egg Substitutes Cow Milks - Processed Goat Milks - Processed Yogurt – Soy

OILS, CONDIMENTS & COOKING

Best Choices/ Allowed	More Best Choices/ Allowed	Continue to Minimize or Avoid
Avocado Oil Bacon Grease Baker's Yeast Baking Powder Baking Soda Butter Coconut Oil Cod Liver Oil Cream of Tartar Flaxseed Oil (but do not cook for cooking) Horseradish Ketchup – Low sugar Lard (Pasturized) Mayonnaise – Natural Mustard Olive Oil Pepper – Black, white, red or Cayenne Pickle Relish Salt – Celtic, Sea Salts Sesame Oil	Vinegar – Balsamic Vinegar – Cider or Red Wine Worcestershire Sauce	Limit your consumption of: Soy Sauce - Any Continue to avoid: Butter Substitutes Canola Oil Margarine – Regular Margarine – Soy Palm Oil Peanut Oil Rice Bran Oil Safflower Oil Salt – Common table varieties Shortening Soybean Oil Sunflower Oil Vegetable Oil – Canola or Corn

SWEETENERS & FLAVORING - Decrease your reliance on all sweeteners!

Best Choices		Continue to Minimize or Avoid
Brown Sugar Carob - Unsweetened Honey Stevia - Herbal sweetener also available in many flavors Vanilla Extract		Agave (use Honey instead) All artificial sweeteners Maple Syrup Molasses White processed sugar - All forms

A special note about these last five food categories:

As these last food groups are filled with many of the food items that we believe are responsible for creating or at very least contributing to the very syndromes that we work to eliminate, we want you to continue to be very cautious about adding significant portions of these foods back into your diet and to watch closely for the signs of any return or worsening of the unwanted symptoms. As we are all very different individuals, we each need to listen to what our own body is telling us about foods that may make us feel worse after being off them for a while. So with that caution in mind, you can try adding back some of these foods in moderate portions and frequency and watch for any regression.

BREAKFAST CEREALS - Applies to both generic & brand name products

Best Choices	Eat Only in Moderation	Continue to Avoid
None are Best Choices!	None are good choices!	All sugared cereals Buckwheat – Kasha Corn flakes Corn grits – White or yellow Cream of rice Cream of wheat Millet – Puffed, cooked Oatmeal or oat bran cereals Rice – Puffed Wheat cereals – All

NUTS & SEEDS – Nuts are fine as snacks and toppings, but eat only in moderation

Best Choices		Continue to Minimize or Avoid
Almonds Almond Butter Cashews Cashew Butter Chestnuts Chia Flaxseed Pistachio Pumpkin Seeds Sesame Seeds		Macadamia Pecans Pine Nuts (Pinion) Sunflower Seeds (kernels or whole) Walnuts **Continue to avoid:** Hazelnuts/ Filberts Peanuts Peanut Butter Soybeans - Roasted or other

GRAINS, FLOURS & NOODLES

Best Choices	Eat Only in Moderation	Continue to Avoid
	* Although these choices are preferred to other options, we suggest you to continue to concentrate on recipes that transition your tastes and lifestyle away from reliance on baked goods and grain foods. Almond Flour Arrowroot Flour Carob Flour Coconut Flour Sweet Potato Flour Tapioca – Pearled & Flour	Amaranth Barley Flour Buckwheat Flour Bulgur Corn Flour – White & yellow Corn Meal – White & yellow Couscous Kamut Macaroni Noodles – Egg, Mung, Rice, Soba, Somen, Spinach, Wheat Oats, Oat Flour & Bran Polenta Quinoa Rice – Brown, White Rice Flour & Bran – Brown, White Rye Flour Soy Flour Spaghetti – Wheat, Spinach Spelt Flour Wheat Flour & Bran Wild Rice

BREADS

Best Choices		Continue to Avoid
None are Best Choices!		Bagels Biscuits – Plain, Butter-milk Cornbread English Muffin – Wheat or White French Bread Oat/Oat Bran Bread Pita Pumpernickel Rice Bran Bread Rye Bread Spelt Bread Tortillas – Corn & Flour Wheat – Whole, Bran, Germ

SNACKS & TREATS

Best Choices	Best Choices (in Moderation)	Continue to Avoid
Celery or carrot sticks Fresh or dehydrated fruit & veggie chunks Jerky, Pemmican (nitrate-free) Nuts from Best Choices list (low-salt & no sugar added) Raisins Sweet potato chips – Natural Tapioca pudding (natural)	Cheese sticks Popcorn (air-popped or with Best Choices oils) - Limit servings to no more than 1 cup (popped)	Candies – Sugared or artificial sweeteners Cookies Corn or Tortilla Chips Crackers (made from grains you should continue to avoid) Graham Crackers Potato Chips Pretzels Rice Cakes

THE FINAL WORD & A REQUEST FOR YOUR HELP

The current medical establishment knows nothing beyond demanding "empirical evidence", being the results of years of highly-expensive research and double-blind testing, in order to accept this type of theory and dietary Protocol. They keep asking me "Why specifically, does this work?", and "Where do all of these theorized imbalances come from?", and "By what exact biological processes does your Protocol work" and all sorts of other questions that, quite frankly, are neither my primary concerns nor issues that we have all the exact answers to at this point in time, as we freely and openly admit. After all; I'm a Naturopath, and no one is exactly burying me in millions of dollars to help me expand this research and my base of case studies.

Unlike them, we're interested in more than empirical evidence, as our sole intent is simply to do our best to create positive results for these kids and adults without a downside. I honestly have no way of knowing at this time how many or what percentage of children and adults who exhibit symptoms both within and outside the Autism Spectrum are even appropriate candidates for this Protocol. But let me just say that wherever I've been able to find my identified commonalities in clinical observation and assessment, the results have been amazingly impressive in the vast majority of cases. Our results over several years are simply far too good to continue to be ignored.

As I have absolutely nothing to "patent" here, I made the decision late in 2009 to disseminate the results of my years of work directly to the public at no cost. I do hold the Copyrights to these writings, however I even grant you the right to make copies of these documents for use by friends, family, neighbors or your doctor - just as long as you don't do so for financial profit. Please don't just copy and give out the "diet" portion alone, as it is not sufficiently informative or compelling without the background of the work.

If you diligently use this Protocol at home or with the assistance of a healthcare provider and start achieving any level of noticeable success, we simply ask and hope that you will do several things in return:

1. First and foremost, tell others! Circulate our information and your personal story of hope to everyone you know in the ADD and Autism communities and post entries on the blogs of research and support groups.

2. If you have not done so already, we encourage everyone to please join our email update list at www.noharmfoundation.org so that we will be able to keep you informed as to new developments

3. Please email us at results@noharmfoundation.org with any feedback regarding your experiences (positive or not) with the dietary Protocol so that we will be able to exponentially build and advance this research. We love to hear all your personal stories and hope to soon also have a blog appearing on our website to serve as an open forum for people to share their experiences with others internationally.

4. Lend your support by making a charitable donation of any affordable size with your check by mail to No Harm Foundation at 150 Rock Point Drive, Suite C, Durango, CO 81301, or with your credit card through the website www.noharmfoundation.org so that this work will continue and gain higher exposure and use. Either method will generate you a donation receipt for tax purposes.

Although it is very important to us that families everywhere are able to access this valuable information and experiment with this program at no direct cost, we want you to consider this to be our "pay it forward" contribution to the wellness of society. The No Harm Foundation is a not-for-profit organization with the missions of advancing the field of natural medicine, preserving health freedom and choice for the public, and broad dissemination of this information about new hope for Autism and other disorders to the general public and medical communities.

The amount of your donation is not important, but simply consider in retrospect what the information was worth to you and to the wellness of your child or other family member and please just do what you can to help us with our continuing efforts to get the word out to countless others and to advance education and effective research on the subject. As resources become available, a portion of this NoHarm charitable fund will also be utilized to subsidize and supply the expenses of families with less than- fortunate circumstances in getting the help they need from our Center and from other healthcare practitioners who choose to join us.

We fully understand any frustration you might feel around the void of localized help available to you at this time, but please know that we have been aggressively trying to attract help and support for this project from the medical communities, a number of Autism organizations and media outlets for several years now, and we have accepted the realization that only by this information directly reaching the attention of the general public will sufficient attention be stimulated and directed towards a form of real progress for the millions of families worldwide that are dealing with these destructive conditions.

Just as soon as possible we will be making available additional written and video training materials that will be able to more extensively explain the science behind my work and provide families more comprehensive instruction on trying to get the best results possible with this dietary Protocol from home until broader professional help is organized. These helpful training materials will be available to you for only modest donations to the No Harm Foundation. Please understand that this is the absolute best we are able to do until such time as enough health practitioners can be trained and join our network so that we can refer one-on-one professional support in your own geographical areas.

You can greatly help this cause in the meantime by sending this message on to any affected families you might know, to therapists and physicians, to any contacts in the media and to anyone else who cares that these syndromes are now needlessly affecting a tragically growing number of our kids. With your help, we'll be able to stimulate enough public and professional awareness so that we can accelerate into a new paradigm of research, prevention and effective care.

Why should people from all across the country and beyond have to travel to visit our Center here in Colorado in order to have access to this safe and inexpensive option, when they should be able to receive simple guidance and support right in their own communities? Amazed and elated parents of our clients are constantly asking us, "Why aren't you able to refer me to practitioners closer to us who are aware of what you're doing?" Our goal is to be able to make that happen very soon.

A large part of our intention in releasing and sharing our findings to date, is to be joined by as many other open-minded practitioners as possible in order to expand this exploration and with it, the number of affected children and families that could be benefiting from this program right now. There's only so much that we can continue to do by ourselves. We need a great number of forward-thinking practitioners, organizations and media outlets who are unwilling to accept the hopeless confines of this prison, and who are willing to listen and join me outside this "box" that has been labeled "Autism".

I also need you – the Moms and Dads out there with affected children to open your minds and hearts and give this a try. This program is safe, and it could be as effective for you as it has been for so many of my clients. There is no down-side, nothing to lose, and so very much to gain. Your child trusts you with their health and well-being. Please always do your best to be worthy of that trust.

Be well,

Shauna

Acknowledgements:

As always, the first thank you's need to go to my Assertive Wellness family; Doris Young, Doug Young, Lori Young, and to Judy Crews Lewis and Rae Lutgen (who are honorary Young's). Some of us are related by blood, but we are all related by our love and commitment to our common goal of helping this important work come to light. These folks are the backbone of everything I do, and I want to thank them for their support, and for oh so patiently dealing with my sometimes incorrigible clients.

Much gratitude goes out to my editor, Lisa Schofield, for once again shaping up my grammar without changing my voice. To Linda Kane for… well… being Linda Kane. To Joe Salama who was incredibly encouraging about this book, and for giving his sage legal advice. To Betty P. for allowing me to share the incredible journey of her son Nick with the world. To Michelle and Keith Norris of Paleo f(x) for giving my work a voice, and to my friends who did not see hide nor hair of me for over six months while I was writing, yet still seem to love me anyway.

In the "no-way-in-the-world-I-could-have-done-it-without-you" category is Glen White for his valuable feedback, for doing such a wonderful job of giving the book its special look, and for always encouraging me to "Trust your gut", which is excellent advice I needed to hear. Oh, and for reminding me to eat once in awhile while I was writing!

More grateful nods go to the good people like our friend Pat Stroh in Tennessee, whose invaluable contributions keep the NoHarm Foundation running. Pat doesn't even have an autistic child, and yet he contributes each and every month so that we can continue to help children the world over! I wish I had room to mention all the wonderful people that have made their donations to NoHarm Foundation; obviously we don't. Just know that you have more than our gratitude: you have our promise that we will use your hard earned funds responsibly.

Speaking of responsible, I must again mention my brother Douglas Young. Not only is he the key component in my "team", he is also the Chairman and Head of The NoHarm Foundation. He keeps the stream of information going out to the public, and there is no one out there fighting harder or more honestly for ASD children. He also cracks me up, and anyone who has ever written a book knows how important that can be…

It is with gratitude mixed with awe that I honor all the families who had already "tried everything," but who were somehow still swinging for the fences for their kids. Despite everything they were willing to trust me and try… just one more thing. To me, that is the face of love and commitment.

Most of all, to "my kids." I may have changed your names for this book, but I remember all of you and could picture each and every one of your faces while I was writing. Thank you for all the intense, wonderful, silly, bizarre, scary and touching moments that I had with you. You have all changed my life. Every single one of you are my legacy, and I can't wait to see all the things; both "common" and "amazing" that you will accomplish with your lives. I just know in my heart that I'll see some of you standing up there on a podium somewhere collecting your well-earned rewards, and I'll be thinking, "Yep. That's my kid."

Seriously, what a ride…

www.ingramcontent.com/pod-product-compliance
Lightning Source LLC
Chambersburg PA
CBHW051850170526
45168CB00001B/47